BEAT THE IRON CRISIS

Iron deficiency is becoming increasingly common amongst young children in the western world. Here is vital information for everyone.

GW00702076

BEAT THE IRON CRISIS

1 in 4 young children are anaemic*

Leonard Mervyn

B.Sc., Ph.D., C.Chem., F.R.S.C.

THORSONS PUBLISHING GROUP

First published 1988

British Library Cataloguing in Publication Data

Mervyn, Leonard
The iron crisis: the major western mineral
deficiency.
1. Iron—Physiological effect
I. Title
612'.3924   QP913.F4

ISBN 0-7225-1578-2

Published by Thorsons Publishers Limited,
Denington Estate, Wellingborough,
Northamptonshire, NN8 2RQ, England

Printed in Great Britain by
Richard Clay Limited, Bungay, Suffolk

1   3   5   7   9   10   8   6   4   2

Contents

Introduction

If the average person were asked to name the minerals they felt were the most important in maintaining health, the chances are that their answer would be iron for the blood and calcium for the bones. Any woman who has been pregnant and under medical supervision will almost certainly have been given these minerals in supplement form whilst she was carrying her child and probably even after giving birth. Iron is the second most abundant metal in the earth's crust (after aluminium), so not surprisingly it is present in all foods that are grown since the soil is the ultimate source of all minerals. Why, then, should many people be at risk of not receiving sufficient of this mineral in their diets?

The reasons are complex and are a combination of iron loss in food refining, differing availabilities from food items, problems in absorption, and the presence of natural inhibiting factors in the normal diet. As the story unfolds it is not difficult to see how the interplay of these factors determines eventually just how much of the iron we eat we can eventually use.

What are the manifestations of iron deficiency? Again if we asked our average individual, the chances are that the answer would be anaemia with all the symptoms that the condition conjures up, namely, paleness, tiredness, easy fatigue, breathlessness, lack of stamina, and eventually apathy and an inability to concentrate. Iron-deficiency anaemia accounts for few deaths, at least here in the western world, but it contributes greatly to the general unhealthy and substandard performance of millions of people. However, new studies have indicated that we must look beyond anaemia alone for the ill effects of iron deficiency, to impaired brain function, mental and physical development, and resistance to infection.

Two recent leading studies in the *British Medical Journal* of 12 April 1986 and in *The Lancet* of 17 January 1987 have reviewed the widespread deficiency of iron in certain communities in the UK and the effect of this deficiency on mental attitudes. 'Happiness is: Iron' is the title of the *British Medical Journal* article that draws attention to iron deficiency in pre-school and school-age children. Not only does lack of the mineral cause poorer results in mental aptitude tests in deficient children, but it also makes them more tense and fearful and hence less happy. The *Lancet* article 'Iron Deficiency—Time for a Community Campaign' reports a disturbingly high incidence of iron-deficiency anaemia amongst children of certain communities in the UK and relates this to a slowing of physical and mental development. The articles beg the question 'should all infants and young children be screened for iron deficiency or is it more beneficial to mount a community campaign to reduce the incidence of the condition as has been carried out in other countries?'

These and other reviews are a sad indictment of modern nutritional practices that allow, in this day and age, iron deficiency to flourish even in the more affluent west. As this book shows, there is no nutritional reason why anyone in this country should be iron deficient, and if the advice in its pages is taken, no one will be. It is now over fifty years since that other great deficiency disease, rickets, was eradicated in the UK. Perhaps we can now hope that the most common mineral deficiency here, and indeed in the world, can follow vitamin D deficiency into the medical history books.

CHAPTER 1

Iron Deficiency and its Manifestations

According to World Health Organization (WHO) figures iron-deficiency anaemia now has a world-wide prevalence of 20 per cent, making it the most common mineral deficiency. Iron-deficiency anaemia may be defined in an individual as a sub-optimal haemoglobin level due to a lack of iron and with no available stores of iron in the body. The WHO define anaemia as a level of haemoglobin below 12g per 100ml blood. In Britain 10 per cent of all women have haemoglobin concentrations below 12g. If these women take oral iron their haemoglobin levels rise. One per cent of British women have less than 8g per 100ml, and at this level the heart output of blood is affected. In these cases medical consultation is essential.

Assessment of iron status

A practical problem in diagnosing anaemia is the wide variation in haemoglobin levels between different normal subjects. If anaemia in an individual is defined as a haemoglobin level two grams below the mean value in a population then there will always be subjects in the population with haemoglobin values within the normal range of the population (in women this is from 12 to 12.6g per 100ml; in men 13.5 to 17.5g per 100ml) but with a depressed formation of haemoglobin in new red blood cells due to a lack of iron. This condition has thus been termed 'iron deficiency without anaemia' or 'latent iron deficiency'.

In actual practice, iron deficiency is defined as a state where there are no available iron stores and with an insufficient supply of iron to the bone marrow and other tissues. Iron-deficiency anaemia is defined as a state when lack of iron has led to a decrease in the haemoglobin level below the average value for the actual population group. Whilst this is 12g per 100ml in non-pregnant women, the figure is set at 13.5g per 100ml in men.

The diagnosis of iron deficiency is still confined to and dependent on laboratory facilities, but in recent years more specific methods have been introduced with greater sensitivity. Nevertheless in a subject with a typical iron deficiency the haemoglobin level is reduced and it is this parameter that is still the most widely used. In addition, the red blood cells are smaller in size than normal and contain less haemoglobin. However, whilst measurement of haemoglobin is the simplest criterion of the extent of iron-deficiency anaemia, the condition can be related to a reduced concentration of iron in the plasma which is bound to the specific protein transferrin. This carrier protein has a reduced saturation level because there is not enough iron to saturate it. Similarly the serum ferritin level is low because this is related to the size of the iron stores. All along the line of haemoglobin degradation and production it is possible to detect low iron levels. For example the bone marrow shows absence of stainable iron (called haemosiderin) and in the specialized cells that remove iron from old haemoglobin (called reticuloendothelial cells) there is less iron. This in turn leads to a reduced number of the cells in the bone marrow that eventually become red blood cells and the ferritin concentration in them is also reduced.

Measurements of all these levels are now possible, and can give a doctor a great deal of information about a patient's iron status. For example, in borderline states with haemoglobin levels within the normal range but with no iron stores, serum ferritin levels are low and there is no stainable iron in the bone marrow smear, whereas the other parameters are within normal range. This condition often happens in old people and one consequence can be a generalized pruritus (or itching). Haemoglobin levels appear adequate but measurement of serum ferritin indicates low serum iron, so without this diagnostic tool an iron deficiency state may be missed. In some cases simple supplementation with oral iron is sufficient to restore serum iron levels and the pruritus is relieved.

Despite all these measurable criteria there are still several sources of error in the laboratory diagnosis of iron deficiency both in clinical practice and in studying epidemiological trends. For example recent infections, recent intake of iron tablets, and the presence of other disorders of the blood can affect the blood parameters that are measured. Hence in certain situations the true prevalence of iron-deficiency anaemia can only be assessed by administering iron supplements in adequate dosage and determining any response. If the haemoglobin and other levels increase on treatment, it can safely be assumed that the original condition was iron-deficiency anaemia.

—The cause and prevalence of iron deficiency—

The most frequent cause of iron deficiency is nutritional: the individual's needs for iron exceed the amount they are absorbing from their diet. In industrialized countries there has been a trend in recent years to reduced expenditure of energy, leading in turn to a reduction in dietary intakes of energy. The relative composition of the diet has changed little, so lower energy intakes also mean less iron intake and hence less uptake. A switch to a higher proportion of dietary energy from fats and refined sugar will also contribute to lower amounts of iron since these foods are devoid of the mineral.

Clinical reasons for iron-deficiency anaemia include increased blood losses from cancers in the gastro-intestinal tract or uterus. Decreased iron absorption can be a feature of gluten sensitivity, lack of stomach acid, and partial or complete gastrectomy (stomach removal). The ways in which iron can be lost from the body are all discussed in greater detail in chapter 3.

In developing countries the amount of iron actually assimilated from the diet is often very low, mainly because of a lack of meat, fish, and vitamin C (ascorbic acid) in the diet, all of which facilitate the absorption of the mineral. Another cause of iron deficiency in these countries is frequent pregnancies with inadequate supplementation that fails to make up all the losses associatated with pregnancy. It is in these countries too that significant losses of iron can arise because of the unwelcome attention of blood-sucking parasites.

There have been a number of studies in various countries of the prevalence of iron deficiency in different population groups. A typical study was that carried out by Dr M. Layrisse and colleagues on 228 Venezuelan peasants who were in apparent good health. The results, reported in the medical journal *Blood* in 1973, were assessed assuming anaemia was present in women with haemoglobin levels of less than 12g per 100ml and in men with levels of less than 13g per 100ml. Of the total number of subjects, 21.5 per cent were judged anaemic; 28.9 per cent were regarded as iron deficient; and 63 per cent absorbed more than 30 per cent of a test dose of ferrous ascorbate, suggesting they were iron depleted. Obviously there was some overlap between the groups.

All is not well, however, in the better-fed western countries. Prevalence studies in the USA in 1976 which measured plasma ferritin levels as well as haemoglobin content of red blood cells indicated that 20 per cent of women and 3 per cent of men had no iron stores in them. Anaemia existed in 8.4 per cent of women and 1.2 per cent of men. Similar figures were found in comparable studies carried out in Sweden.

The Swedish experience is a salutary lesson to us all. A study carried out in 1965 indicated that between 25 and 30 per cent of women of child-bearing age were anaemic. In a follow-up study carried out some ten years later, Dr L. Hallberg and his colleagues were able to report in the *Bulletin of the World Health Organization* (1979) that the incidence of iron-deficient anaemia had dropped dramatically to 6–7 per cent. What were the reasons?

The increased use of oral contraceptives during the intervening period would have caused decreased menstrual blood losses since usage of the 'Pill' gives rise to a thinner uterine endometrium. The fortification of all types of flour was increased from 30 to 75mg per kg. Both prescribed and non-prescribed iron preparations increased to a total intake of more than 17,000kg, equivalent to 5.8mg of the mineral per head daily, a figure more than five times that in the UK. Vitamin C sales also increased, with the result that the iron preparations and iron in the food were better absorbed.

In the publication quoted, the authors discussed the relative importance of the various factors thought to contribute to the increased iron uptake by the population, particularly by women. They concluded that iron supplementation, prescribed or otherwise, accounted for a reduction of 10 per cent in the prevalence of anaemia; the higher rate of fortification of flour contributed a further 7-8 per cent reduction. On the other side of the coin, 4 men out of 347 persons who were screened were found on biochemical measurement to have iron stores greatly in excess of normal.

If we look at other communities in the western world it becomes obvious that there is no room for complacency in the incidence of iron-defiency anaemia. In the UK, for example, we do not see today the staggering incidence reported in poor families of Aberdeen in the 1930s (Davidson *et al.*, *British Medical Journal* (1935)), when all the pregnant women (about 800) were below or at 10g haemoglobin per 100ml blood and two-thirds of non-pregnant women had levels below 11.3g per 100ml. During the same period Dr H. M. Mackay reported in *Archives of Diseases of Childhood* (1933) that 582 out of a total 594 infants in London had haemoglobin levels lower than normal value of 11.3g per 100ml expected.

These were poverty-stricken communities, but modern research has indicated comparable figures today in many cities of the world where similar poverty exists. In the UK, iron deficiency is less common than formerly but still exists. One report by Dr P. C. Elwood in 1968 (*Proceedings of the Nutrition Society*) found that out of 1,080 women in South Wales, 100 of them had haemoglobin levels of less than 12g per 100ml.

Although women in their reproductive years are the population sector most likely to suffer iron-deficiency anaemia, infants and children are also affected, and for the following reasons:

1. Prolonged milk feeding
   Both breast-fed and artificially fed infants may be kept too long on milk alone with no supplementary iron and iron-containing food.
2. Low birth weight
   Normally at birth a full-term baby has a haemoglobin level of about 17g per 100ml blood. After birth the red blood cells are broken down so that by the sixth to eighth week the haemoglobin falls to about 11g per 100ml blood. The iron released by this natural process is stored in the liver for later utilization during the period of milk feeding. Once weaning starts, the haemoglobin rises because of increased intakes of

iron and by the end of nine months should reach about 13g per 100ml blood.

Premature babies and those of full-term but low birth weight (e.g. twins) have a small blood volume and thus smaller stores of iron to tide them over the milk only feeding period. In addition, their rate of growth is greater and so their demand for iron is increased.

3. Anaemia in the mother
When the mother suffers from nutritional iron-deficiency anaemia she is less able to pass on adequate amounts of the mineral to the foetus, which will be born with low stores.

4. Infant infections and malabsorption
The common infections of infancy and childhood are known to suppress the formation of red blood cells by the bone marrow, so anaemia is inevitable. Those who have an intolerance to gluten may develop iron-deficiency anaemia because of an inability to absorb adequate amounts of the mineral.

————Symptoms and prevention in infants————

The symptoms of iron-deficiency anaemia are not easily recognized in babies and small children apart from a general decrease in general healthiness and vitality. These are not specific, however, and before treatment is started with iron, measurement of blood parameters is essential to confirm the diagnosis. Before this stage is reached, however, there are certain measures that can be taken to prevent the onset of iron deficiency in infants. Prevention must start before birth by ensuring that pregnant women have adequate iron in their diets, supplemented with oral iron when necessary. Infections in infants must be treated promptly to avoid suppression of the bone marrow. Weaning with iron-rich broth, minced meat, vegetable purées, and easily digested sources of iron is essential from the age of 4–6 months. In low birth weight infants small amounts of iron may be administered as a supplement from three months of age. If anaemia has developed, treatment by dietary improvement alone cannot be relied upon to cure the anaemia and supplementation becomes essential. Usually a daily amount of 6mg iron per kg body weight is taken in a well-diluted form.

──────Clinical features of anaemia in adults──────

Reduced levels of haemoglobin mean a lower oxygen-carrying capacity of the red blood cells, so many signs and symptoms of iron-deficiency anaemia relate to reduced oxygen availability. When the transport of oxygen by the blood is insufficient to meet the needs of the body, symptoms arise. This need for oxygen is related to physical activity, so a person leading a sedentary life may have a moderate degree of anaemia yet be free of obvious symptoms. Once they take unaccustomed exercise, however, symptoms will arise. Any significant degree of anaemia is always associated with an inability to make sustained physical effort. When the anaemia develops very slowly, the individual may gradually and unwittingly reduce physical activity to a lower level and so be unaware of the anaemia. A housewife with a haemoglobin level of less than 7.5g per 100ml blood may find she can undertake her normal housework but takes longer to do it.

How severely the individual reacts to iron-deficiency anaemia is dependent not only on the degree of anaemia but on the rapidity of its development. Common symptoms are general fatigue and lassitude, breathlessness on exertion, giddiness, dimness of vision, headache, insomnia, pallor of the skin, palpitation, anorexia (loss of appetite) and indigestion, tingling and 'pins and needles' in the fingers and toes.

Physical signs include pallor of the mucous or wet membranes: e.g. the normal healthy pink membranes inside the eyelids are replaced by pale colourless ones. Often the usual pink flare spreading from the half-moons of the fingernails is missing. In iron-deficiency anaemia, the tongue and lower lip lose the pink colour associated with a normal haemoglobin level. These simple signs, which anyone can observe, have been used as a cheap screening programme in rural areas of India. Drs S. Ghosh and M. Mohan reported a successful campaign using these criteria in *The Lancet* (1978) and claimed that in their Indian study 100 per cent of patients with haemoglobin levels of less than 6g per 100ml blood and 67 per cent of those with levels between 6 and 9g per 100ml were correctly identified. The rate of success with children was even higher, but the failures in adult patients were associated with lips discoloured by tobacco and betel-nut chewing.

The shape of the nails can be indicative of iron-deficiency

anaemia. There is a condition called koilonychia which appears in various stages. First there is brittleness and dryness, but as the anaemia develops there is flattening and thinning of the nails. Finally the nails become concave and spoon-shaped. At this stage, anaemia is virtually guaranteed.

An observation first reported in 1908 by Dr W. Osler has aroused interest in anaemia diagnosis in modern times. He reported that a blueness of the white of the eye (the sclera) was associated with iron deficiency. Drs L. Kalra, A. N. Hamlyn, and B. J. M. Jones of Wordsley Hospital, Stowbridge, in the UK tested Osler's hypothesis on 169 adult in-patients. The colour of the sclera was assessed by three different observers. The presence of anaemia was indicated by a haemoglobin level of less than 12g per 100ml blood for premenopausal women and less than 12.5g per 100ml for postmenopausal women and for men.

Twenty-eight per cent of the patients had definite or striking blueness of their sclera, and of these 85 per cent had iron deficiency. Conversely, 87 per cent of the patients with iron deficiency, both men and women, had blue in their sclera. These were all in-patients. A follow-up study (The Lancet [1987]) on 1,829 consecutive out-patients (31.9 per cent men an. td 68.1 per cent women) confirmed the earlier findings. Eighty-three per cent of patients with blue in their sclera had evidence of past or present iron deficiency. Only seven women who exhibited blue in their sclera were found to have iron deficiency.

The reasons for the phenomena are purely hypothetical. Since iron is needed for the synthesis of collagen (the protein that binds cells and tissues together), iron deficiency may lead to thin sclera through which the larger blood vessels can be seen, making the whites of the eye appear blue. The authors suggest that the presence of a bluish tinge to the sclera should alert both patient and doctor to a possible underlying iron deficiency.

—Effects of anaemia not related to haemoglobin—
We have seen that the negative effects of iron deficiency can be ascribed mainly to the anaemia and the impaired delivery of oxygen to the tissues. The effect upon the iron-containing enzymes in various parts of the body is also significant. This has been confirmed by experiments on rats which were iron deficient. Their

working capacity was reduced dramatically even though the anaemia, in terms of haemoglobin content, was mild. The negative effect of the deficiency was not due to the anaemia but to lack of iron-containing tissue enzymes that function in the energy-producing processes of the tissues. In any type of fatigue where these enzymes are deficient or lacking the amount of lactic acid in the blood increases. This is because the body is incapable of burning this acid off further to carbon dioxide and water, which is a very important energy-producer. The experimental rats all had high levels of blood lactic acid (C. A. Finch *et al.*, *Journal of Clinical Investigation* [1976]).

These studies were confirmed in human beings who were iron deficient. They too had a greatly reduced work capacity even though the degree of anaemia appeared mild because haemoglobin levels were only slightly low. Nevertheless, when treated with iron, these people had a greatly improved work capacity that could not be totally accounted for by the moderate rise in haemoglobin.

Iron-containing and iron-dependent enzymes such as cytochromes, peroxidase, catalase, and metalloflavoprotein enzymes which are all concerned with oxygen usage and energy production are depleted in iron-deficiency anaemia. Children who are severely iron deficient often suffer from restlessness and irritability and these symptoms can be related to increased levels of stimulant substances called catecholamines in their bodies. When they are treated with iron, the catecholamines drop to normal levels and their behaviour returns to normal. Recent experiments with rats have confirmed this finding in children and the mechanism of how iron deficiency produces these symptoms appears to be mediated through the thyroid gland (E. Pollit and R. L. Leibel, *Iron Deficiency, Brain Biochemistry and Behaviour* [Raven Press, 1981]).

Iron and mental development

Although the ill effects of chronic iron-deficiency anaemia are well recognized, the importance of iron extends far beyond its role as a constituent of haemoglobin. Recently, studies have switched to the effects of lack of iron on functions not related to red blood cells. Animal studies have shown that irrespective of the anaemia, iron deficiency produces defects in muscle and impairs the normal functioning of the white blood cells. More importantly, however, there is now growing evidence that iron deficiency has an adverse effect on brain function. When rats were made deficient in the mineral there was disturbed enzyme activity in their brains, leading to lack of production of brain substances essential for memory and other functions. The learning ability of rats was severely curtailed when they were iron deficient.

Confirmation of these studies in human beings has come from several observations that iron deficiency in children, with or without anaemia, is associated with abnormalities of behaviour and mental performance. These functions improved when the children were treated with iron.

A typical study was that by F. A. Oski and A. S. Honig, reported in the *Journal of Paediatrics* (1978). They investigated 24 iron-deficient anaemic children aged from 9 to 26 months. Twelve children were given intramuscular iron and twelve received an inactive placebo. Tests of mental development and behaviour were carried out and assessed before the injection and five to eight days later. Improvements were found in all children given iron, but those given the placebo were no better after the injection than before it. Other benefits in the iron-treated group included a more responsive attitude to their environment.

A similar study carried out in Guatemala and reported in the *Journal of Paediatrics* (1982) by Dr B. Lozoff and her colleagues found that children with iron-deficiency anaemia had lower scores than other children in tests of mental development. The deficient children were also less responsive and appeared more tense and fearful. One week's treatment with oral iron supplements did not cause any improvement in the results but later studies suggested that the period of therapy was too short to be effective.

As a follow-up to the trial mentioned above, Dr F. A. Oski and colleagues studied babies aged 9 to 12 months who were iron deficient but not anaemic. The tests that measured mental performance gave better results after all the babies received intramuscular iron injections. Improvement was seen as soon as one week after injection. This mode of administering iron will build up iron levels far quicker than the oral route, which is why response was so much more rapid.

The validity of such studies was confirmed world-wide in such widespread countries as Chile, Java, Egypt, and the UK. A group of 15-month-old Chilean children deficient in iron were reported by Dr T. Walter and colleagues to achieve low scores in their tests of mental development before iron therapy; the scores increased dramatically after it. It did, however, take 11 days of iron replacement therapy before improvement could be measured.

Professor E. Pollitt of the University of Texas reported two selective results from studies on children sponsored by the Food, Nutrition, and Poverty Programme of the United Nations University at the eighth annual meeting of the International Nutritional Anaemia Consultation Group held in Bali in late 1984. Both reports on the cognitive effects of iron-deficiency anaemia, from double-blind (i.e. neither subject nor doctor is aware who is being treated with iron or with the placebo) iron-nutritional clinical trials, indicated that body iron status among school-age children correlated strongly with educational achievement and efficiency in problem solving.

The first study was carried out in Central Java and focused on 119 children with an average age of 10.8 years. Seventy-eight children had iron-deficiency anaemia; the other 41 were iron replete. Forty-three of those who were anaemic and 16 of the non-anaemic children were treated with ferrous sulphate tablets at a dosage of 10mg per kg body weight daily for five months. All the remaining children received a placebo. They were all assessed using an abbreviated version of the standard achievement test (mathematics, biology, social science, and language) already in use in the school system. The results were as follows. Before iron therapy, non-anaemic children achieved consistently and significantly higher achievement scores than the anaemic children. After therapy, the achievement scores of iron-treated anaemic children and placebo-treated non-anaemic children remained the same. The achievement scores of anaemic children were higher after iron treatment than before it and also higher than the placebo-treated subjects. However, the scores of the non-anaemic children were still significantly better than those of the iron-treated anaemic children. This would suggest that five months therapy was not sufficient to achieve the iron status of non-anaemic children or that some other deficiency may exacerbate that of iron. In malnutrition, it is rare to find one isolated micronutrient deficiency.

These children were all tested in academic subjects, and the rapid improvement after treatment would suggest that the deficit was either in recall or performance rather than learning. This study, like the following one, was reported in *The Lancet* (19 January 1985).

The second comprehensive study was carried out in a semi-urban community of Cairo, Egypt. Sixty-eight children (average age 9.5 years) were chosen from an original 203 and of those chosen, 28 were defined on the basis of haemoglobin content and ferritin concentration of the blood as iron anaemic; the other 40 were regarded as iron replete on the same criteria. For four months, 18 of the iron-deficient and 19 of the iron-replate subjects received daily 50mg of iron orally as ferrous sulphate. All of the other children received placebos.

In this trial, the test was a problem-solving one of matching a figure on a card with a similar figure amongst six cards five of which displayed a variant of the original figure. The time taken to match correctly was measured and the errors made before a perfect match was achieved were also noted. In this way efficiency and impulsivity could be compared.

The efficiency, speed of response, and accuracy of the matching were all faster in the non-anaemic than in the iron-deficient children before iron supplementation. After iron was given, the efficiency of iron-treated anaemic children was significantly greater than that of children treated with the placebo. Hence it can be concluded that the children who were originally anaemic and treated with iron became faster and more accurate in their responses than did those who received only the placebo. There were no significant differences between the iron- and placebo-treated iron-replete children, which indicates that extra iron in a well-nourished child is unlikely to improve mental performance. The efficiency score of the iron-treated anaemic children was similar to that of the untreated non-anaemic controls.

Professor Pollitt concludes that both sets of data support the hypothesis that iron deficiency adversely affects the learning and problem-solving capacity of school-age children.

In a review paper published in 1986 by the *American Journal of Clinical Nutrition,* Professor Pollitt went further in assessing the relationship between iron deficiency and behavioural development in infants and pre-school children. The previous studies looked at children receiving education, but what happens in the years leading up to the first school?

Professor Pollitt studied 50 Guatemalan children in the age range three to six years, 25 of whom were iron deficient and anaemic and 25 who were iron replete. Performance before and after oral iron therapy was measured in memory and learning tasks and in maintaining attention and resistance to distraction. Oral iron therapy was continued for 11 to 12 weeks. All infants with iron deficiency, whether anaemic or not, scored lower than the iron-replete ones in these tests (called collectively the Bayley Scale of Neonatal Development), but there was no association between iron deficiency and the development of physical abilities. After iron therapy, the mental development scores neared those of non-anaemic infants. In terms of problem solving, the institution of iron supplements increased the ability of the anaemic subjects to solve problems. Before iron was given, however, those with iron deficiency were less likely to pay attention to relevant clues in problem-solving situations.

Along with improvement in learning and problem solving induced by iron in iron-deficient babies, toddlers, and schoolchildren there also appeared to be changes in mental attitude. Iron reduced the tenseness and fearfulness noted in iron deficiency, with the result that the subjects who responded appeared to be less unhappy than they were before treatment. This criterion alone may make zealous mothers reach for the iron to make their charges happier, but unless the unhappiness was related to the mineral deficiency in the first place, supplementation is unlikely to help.

In a recent study nearer home paediatricians from Sorrento Maternity Hospital in Birmingham concluded that iron deficiency in toddlers should be hunted out and treated as it may slow down their cognitive development. The trial was stimulated by the finding that iron-deficiency anaemia is very common in pre-school children in the catchment area of this hospital and paediatricians had noted that the anaemic children appeared to develop slowly. What was not clear was whether the anaemia and slow development were just two symptoms of an underprivileged environment or if the iron deficiency actually causes the delay in development. The study, reported by Dr M. A. Auckett and colleagues in the journal *Archives of Disease in Childhood* (1986), seemed to confirm similar ones carried out elsewhere and discussed above.

The trial was the double-blind type on iron supplementation in toddlers living in an underprivileged area of the inner city of Birmingham. Four hundred and seventy children aged 17 to 19 months were screened for anaemia and iron deficiency at child health clinics in central Birmingham. About 26 per cent of them were found to be anaemic, with haemoglobin levels of less than 11g per 100ml blood. Eight were so anaemic as to require immediate therapy. The remainder were invited to attend an anaemia clinic at the hospital where growth was measured and psychomotor (i.e. concerning physical activity associated with mental processes) development was assessed using the Denver Screening Test.

The children were divided into two groups, one receiving 24mg of iron plus 10mg vitamin C daily and the other a matching syrup containing only 10mg vitamin C. After two months on either treatment (which was supervised), the children were assessed again using the Denver Screening Test.

Any average child in the 17-19 months age range should gain six new skills on the Denver test in two months, and this was the criterion on which the trial was based. Fifteen of the 48 children taking iron supplements achieved this figure, which represents an average rate of development, but only six out of the 49 control children did so. In addition, the iron-treated children gained weight significantly faster than did those on vitamin C alone.

The investigating doctors say that the difference in psychomotor development and weight gain between the two groups is significant and suggest there is a direct relationship between these two criteria and iron status. They do emphasize, however, that iron deficiency is unlikely to be the only factor in slow psychomotor development as a number of children were still below average in recent testing despite increases in haemoglobin levels. It is, however, a factor that can be easily identified and treated and they suggest that a screening test for anaemia be included in health surveillance programmes for children in underprivileged areas.

Iron deficiency in children

Iron deficiency in childhood is common even in socially advantaged populations, but more so in those who are socially deprived according to Dr F. A. Oski writing in *Pediatr. Clin. North America* in 1985. This conclusion has now been confirmed in a study reported by Dr P. Ehrhardt in the *British Medical Journal* of January 1986, who measured the blood haemoglobin and/or serum ferritin levels in most of 778 Bradford, UK, children over a six-month period. All of the children were in the pre-school age range of 6 months to 4 years and came from different ethnic groups. Of the total, 513 were white and 265 were of Asian ethnic origin; together they accounted for approximately 6 per cent of the children in this age range residing in the Bradford Health District. The proportions of boys to girls were similar in both ethnic groups and compared well with those in the community as a whole, so the results were presented irrespective of sex.

One hundred and eighty of the children (mainly white) had no blood tests performed on them because they were admitted for gastro-intestinal problems, so in all the diagnostic categories there was a tendency to more complete studies in the children from the Asian ethnic minority. Hence two-thirds of them were studied fully, which could reflect a greater willingness by the admitting doctors to recognize the possibility of iron deficiency in the Asian children.

Out of a total of 598 children whose blood haemoglobins were measured almost 25 per cent (147) were anaemic, and almost 33 per cent (131) of the 400 children whose serum ferritin was measured were iron deficient. Both findings were more common in children from the Asian ethnic minority. At the same time, both anaemia and iron deficiency were more prevalent in those children from the poorer sections of the community studied. Such deficiencies were not confined to the Asian ethnic minority children, but were also found in about one-quarter of the white children.

The results, according to Dr Ehrhardt, justify a routine full blood count in young children admitted to hospital, whatever their ethnic origin, to assess them for anaemia and iron deficiency. He calls for a community campaign to prevent iron deficiency similar to the Stop Rickets Campaign of over fifty years ago. Such a campaign has its precedents. In the United States, e.g., the Women, Infants, and Children (WIC) programme of supplementary feeding has reduced the incidence of childhood iron deficiency according to a report in the *Journal of Paediatrics* (1985).

A successful strategy was (i) an iron-fortified formula given to infants up to the age of one year; (ii) iron-fortified cereal and vitamin C-fortified juice from 6 months to 1 year of age; and (iii) milk, iron-fortified cereal, eggs, vitamin C-fortified juice, cheese, and dried beans from 1 to 5 years of age. At the same time it was suggested that breast-feeding should be encouraged, as should a wider consumption of orange juice containing vitamin C to improve the absorption of iron from the food.

Iron deficiency in the elderly

Iron deficiency has been found to be the commonest cause of anaemia encountered in the elderly, both in the general population and in hospitalized patients. The results of typical studies are presented in Table 1. The criterion for anaemia was a haemoglobin level below 12.0g per 100ml in females and 13.0g per 100ml in males, except in the 1968 study, when 10g per 100ml was chosen in both sexes. This is why the incidence of anaemia in this study is so much lower than in the others.

The cause of this high incidence of anaemia is not known with certainty, but poor iron absorption due to lack of stomach acid (achlorhydria) and structural changes induced by age in the intestinal iron-absorbing cells and enzymes are thought to contribute. A recent study by Dr J. J. M. Marx reported in the journal *Blood* in 1979 has suggested that absorption of iron in the elderly is not impaired, but that they do have a reduced capacity to retain the mineral. His figures indicate that only 66 per cent of absorbed iron was retained in the elderly, compared to 91 per cent of that in young adults.

One other significant effect of iron deficiency in the elderly, apart from obvious anaemia, has been reported by dermatologist Dr G. Auckland, among others, in the UK. One of the commonest

Table 1 Anaemia and iron deficiency in the elderly

Report	Age (years)	No. of subjects	Incidence of anaemia %	Incidence of iron-deficient anaemia in total anaemic subjects %
The Lancet (1958)	65 or over	156	41.0	94
British Medical Journal (1967)	60 or over	100	33.0	10
Gerontologica Clinica (1968)	65 or over	2,700	6.4	67
International Journal of Vitamin Nutrition and Research (1973)	65 or over	93	62.4	—
Journal of the American Geriatric Society (1975)	60 or over	484	31.0	49

skin problems in later life is generalized pruritus (itching). Even though the haemoglobin level may be normal, a deficiency of serum iron can lead to this distressing complaint. Once the presence of low iron stores has been established, a course of iron therapy to replenish then often clears the pruritus completely. Even without blood measurements, it is worth while for any elderly person suffering from pruritus to take iron supplementation to eradicate the complaint.

——Iron deficiency and resistance to infection——

There is some evidence that anaemia may lower resistance to, or recovery from, infections. Some forty years ago it was reported by H. M. M. MacKay *et al.* in *Archives of Disease in Childhood* (1946) that in one nursery of children with relatively low haemoglobin levels, iron therapy was accompanied by a reduction in the absence rate due to infective disease of about 25 per cent. Many years later a Swedish doctor, M. Bondestam and colleages found that Swedish children who were found to be unduly susceptible to infection had lower serum iron levels than comparable healthy children (*Acta Paediatrica Scandinavica* [1985]).

Amongst less advantaged children, giving a nutritional supplement of iron produced an impressive reduction in infectious disease in a study of rural Colombian children reported by J. N. Lukens in *American Journal of Diseases of Childhood* (1975). In the USA it has been established that community-wide feeding programmes can virtually eliminate iron deficiency and reduce infections (*Paediatrics* [1985]). However, in the UK a DHSS report in 1980 entitled 'Inequalities in Health' claimed that children from higher economic groups suffered less mortality and illness than those from poorer groups. An important difference between the two groups was the higher nutritional status, including that of iron, in the better-off group.

On the other hand, it is known that iron is a growth factor for many micro-organisms, including those causing infection, and it has been suggested that iron therapy can reactivate pre-existing infections. For example, in a study carried out in East Africa (Dr O. Higashi *et al.* [1976]) an increase in malarial attacks was reported when adult patients with iron-deficiency anaemia were treated with iron. This may have been the result of increased production of immature red blood cells (called reticulocytes), however, rather than of a direct potentiating effect of the administered iron on the growth of malarial parasites.

These conflicting results may be due to the extent of availability of iron from the host to the invading micro-organism. The host needs the iron to maintain their own immune system, which protects against infection. The mineral is necessary to stimulate the response by body cells and also to ensure that the white blood cells operate at maximum efficiency. At the same time the body needs to prevent iron uptake by the infective bacteria. Hence whilst iron deficiency may increase the host's ability to withhold iron from bacteria, this advantage may be outweighed by impairment of the immune system.

Normal iron balance therefore seems to achieve a compromise in which iron is not readily accessible to invading micro-organisms yet is present in sufficient quantity to allow the host's immune system to function optimally. The balance of evidence would now indicate that the benefits of preventing or treating iron deficiency by fortification of foods or by oral therapy outweighs any risks of exacerbating an infection.

————The advantages of iron deficiency————

We have seen that one possible benefit of a mild iron deficiency is a reduced propensity to infection, but there may be others. For example an epidemiological study reported in 1974 by Dr P. C. Elwood *et al.* related mortality over a three-year period to the red blood cell content of blood, known as the haematocrit. In 18,740 women they found evidence of a small increase in mortality in anaemic subjects but a distinct increase in mortality in subjects with a high haematocrit, i.e. over 46 per cent. This figure represents the percentage volume of the red blood cells in 100ml whole blood. While in the more anaemic women a higher than expected proportion of deaths was due to cancers, this was probably accounted for by the fact that some forms of cancer result in anaemia rather than the converse. What was clear, however, was a distinctly reduced chance of death from cardio-vascular disease in those who were anaemic compared to those with high haematocrit values.

Another benefit associated with mild anaemia is that there is a more efficient formation of anastomoses between blood-vessels. If a blood-vessel is blocked, usually by a thrombosis, other blood-vessels irradiate from one side of the blockage to join up with those from the other side to form an effective by-pass. The ability to form these anastomoses determines the rate of recovery from a thrombosis. Although a mild anaemia confers these benefits there is no evidence to suggest that better anastomoses form with a more severe anaemia. The speed of formation of anastomoses and their persistence can be life-saving in cases of thrombosis of the heart and brain.

Dr Elwood and others have also examined the relationship between anaemia and the level of blood fats (*Lancet* [1970] and *Pathology* [1973] respectively). A total of 4,070 adult women were studied, of whom 124 had haemoglobin levels below 10.5g per 100ml blood. Their mean cholesterol level was only 211mg per 100ml compared to random samples of non-anaemic women, who had a level of 241mg per 100ml. This difference is highly significant since raised blood serum cholesterol is believed to be one of the most important risk factors in the development of coronary heart disease.

A high blood haematocrit value will effectively increase the viscosity of the blood, i.e. make it thicker. An increased viscosity has been linked to increased chances of coronary thrombosis by a number of studies including G. E. Burch *et al.*, *American Journal of Medicine* (1962) and S. Eisenberg, *Circulation* (1966). These researchers and others have evidence that a raised haematocrit is more likely to precede a coronary attack than is a lower one, so here again, a mild anaemia may be a protective factor against thrombosis.

A high haematocrit means higher viscosity blood which is harder to circulate through the blood-vessel system, so that the blood-pressure must increase accordingly to maintain blood flow. This logical sequence of events has been confirmed by Dr G. Tibblin and colleagues (*American Heart Journal* [1966]), who found that blood viscosity is higher in subjects with early high blood-pressure disease than in those with normal blood-pressure. Haematocrits were not measured, but high viscosity by inference means a high percentage of red blood cells in the blood. A lower haematocrit is more conducive to lower blood-pressure.

These studies and observations of his own have led Dr J. L. Sullivan of the V. A. Medical Center, Charleston, USA to propose that one reason why women have a lower incidence of coronary heart-disease is their regular loss of blood in the menstrual flow during their child-bearing years. This loss of blood leads to iron depletion, which in turn protects against coronary heart-disease. Once women reach the menopause and menstrual flow stops, iron stores increase and the incidence of coronary heart-disease approaches that of men of similar age groups. Other conditions in which iron depletion and low incidence of coronary heart disease may be associated include Third World diets; blood loss through parasites; blood donation in excessive quantities; high fish-oil levels in the diet; and long-term use of aspirin and similar anti-thrombosis drugs.

How may lack of iron produce these beneficial effects? Iron depletion is known to decrease tissue injury induced by toxins; it may cause improved anti-oxidant effects resulting in greater protection potential for the heart; and it may be associated with decreased low-density lipoprotein cholesterol, the undesirable cholesterol carrier in the blood. Removing excessive iron with chelating agents improves the survival rates of rats with induced cardiac arrest, and this is akin to a condition of iron depletion.

It must be stressed that all these observations indirectly support the hypothesis that iron depletion may protect against coronary heart-disease, but direct proof is lacking because of the difficulty in creating meaningful clinical trials in human beings. Perhaps the traditional medical treatment of bleeding patients which in itself induced a rapid anaemia had something to recommend it at least in certain conditions.

CHAPTER 2

–Providing Our Needs–

Iron is an essential trace mineral for man and all animal life. It has the chemical symbol Fe, derived from the latin name *ferrum*. In the earth's crust it is present in amounts second only to aluminium, the world's most abundant metal.

Iron does not occur in nature as the free metal but is always combined with other elements like oxygen, with which it forms oxides. There is a wide variety of oxides varying in colour from red to brown to black, and it is this property that makes iron oxide pigments very useful as natural colouring agents for tablets, capsules, and some foods.

When iron is combined with other elements to form mineral salts or with natural materials like protein to form organic complexes it can exist as two forms known as ferrous and ferric compounds. Ferric iron is the oxidized form of ferrous iron. Conversely, ferrous iron is the reduced form of ferric iron. It is the fact that iron can exist in these two interconvertible states that contributes to its functions as an essential trace mineral in human metabolism.

It is of paramount importance that the existence of the two types of iron is understood from the start, because each has its role to play. Iron in the earth's crust is mainly in the ferric form, and so this is how it appears in plants that grow in the soil. Ferric iron complexes tend to be less water-soluble than ferrous iron complexes, so when we eat foodstuffs containing ferric iron, less of the mineral is likely to be absorbed. We shall see later how other constituents of the diet, notably vitamin C, can reduce ferric iron in food to ferrous iron, so solubilizing the mineral and improving its absorption.

As a general rule, in its major role in human metabolism, iron exists in the ferrous state. In its transport and storage within the body, iron exists in its more stable ferric state. We have seen that in foods of plant origin it is also in the ferric state, but in animal-derived foods it tends to be stabilized by protein in the ferrous state. The inter-conversion between ferrous and ferric forms thus assumes importance in the mechanisms by which iron is presented to the body in the diet, is absorbed, is transported within the body, and is eventually excreted. In its functioning it acts exclusively in the ferrous state.

Iron in foodstuffs

Iron is present in virtually all types of foods, but there are two different kinds in the diet, haem iron and non-haem iron. Haem iron can be regarded as exclusive to foods of animal, fish, and fowl origin; non-haem iron is also present to a small extent in these foods, but is the only type of iron found in foods of vegetable origin. As we shall see later, the type of iron in the diet determines the efficiency of absorption of the mineral, but once it is assimilated into the bloodstream any differences cease to exist.

The amount of iron in the same foodstuffs can vary over a wide range of values, partly because of differences in the iron content of soils, which can vary more than a hundredfold. The results of one study carried out in the USA indicated this when several samples of particular vegetables were assayed for their iron content. In each case the highest and lowest figures are shown in parts per million: snap beans 277-10; cabbage 94-20; lettuce 516-19; tomatoes 1,938-1; spinach 1,584-91. The figures illustrate that if any of these sources is the sole supplier of iron in the diet, the correct intake is very much a matter of chance. They emphasize the importance of a mixed and varied diet, taking vegetables from a wide variety of sources to ensure that lack of the mineral in one may be compensated by enough from another. Happily, in this age of fast transport it is no longer necessary to rely on local produce and a variety of vegetables can be eaten from places far afield, even other countries. Iron is a stable mineral, so no loss is incurred during delays between farm and kitchen.

Why should the iron content of vegetables be so variable? The reason is that iron availability to plants is determined both by factors that affect the ability of the soil to supply the mineral and by the factors that affect the plant's ability to utilize the nutrient that is supplied. This means that even if ample iron is present in the soil, uptake by the plant may not be efficient because of interfering factors that are usually environmental.

For effective uptake and utilization by the plant, the iron must be present in a soluble or ionized form. This is determined to a large extent by the acidity of the soil. A highly acid soil keeps the iron in solution, and hence the mineral is available for absorption. As a soil becomes more alkaline the iron is less soluble and the chances of sufficient uptake of the mineral by the plant decrease. The process of liming a highly acid soil is often carried out to prevent excessive intake of toxic minerals that can harm the plant, but the practice may at the same time halt or decrease iron assimilation. The secret is to try to maintain the soil between a medium and slightly acid state so that sufficient iron for a healthy plant is absorbed, but not enough to kill the plant.

It has been calculated that one-third of the world's land is calcareous, i.e. has a high content of calcium (or lime), and this is a common cause of iron deficiency in plants. At the other end of the scale, peaty soils, which are highly acidic, should cause very efficient uptake of iron, but the presence of interfering minerals like manganese, copper, and zinc can have a deleterious effect. The professional farmer knows about his soil and acts accordingly to produce good yields of crops, but the amateur gardener should be aware of these potential problems if he is to produce healthy plants replete in iron.

Iron deficiency in plants produces a condition called chlorosis, and this is also an old name for an iron-deficiency anaemia that is prevalent amongst young women. Typical symptoms of chlorosis in plants are yellowing of the veins in young leaves; stems become short and slender, and whilst buds remain alive, they do not thrive. Never forget that ultimately all minerals come from the soil; and any deficiency of iron in the plants we eat will eventually be reflected in our own deficient intake.

Refined and whole foods

Although many food items are refined and processed to produce foodstuffs that may appear to be more attractive and hence more acceptable to the consumer, the price paid is a serious decrease in the content of iron and other minerals. The simplest example is flour. Wholemeal flour is produced by grinding the wholewheat grains, so retaining all the nutrients and micronutrients of the original wheat. The iron content of this flour is 4mg per 100g. White flour, on the other hand, is produced by first removing the bran and wheatgerm of the wholegrain and grinding down the resulting white endosperm. The iron content of this flour is only 1.5mg per 100g, representing a loss of 37.5 per cent. Some iron is put back into white flour under present legislation, but the case does illustrate how losses of iron can occur by simple refining processes. Perhaps it is not surprising when we consider that the bulk of the iron in a wholewheat grain is in the bran and wheatgerm parts and it is these that are removed in the production of white flour. Both ingredients are incorporated into animal feeds, which is one reason why farm animals on the whole are probably better fed than we are.

As a general rule, refined cereals will tend to have lower iron contents than the natural grains from which they were derived. It is, however, worth bearing in mind that both wheat bran and wheatgerm are rich sources of iron (12.9 and 10.0mg per 100g respectively), which is an added bonus to those who take these foodstuffs essentially as a source of extra dietary fibre. In recent debates on the attributes or otherwise of high bran intakes none of the protagonists seems to have pointed out that this nutrient also supplies significant quantities of all the essential minerals. In view of this, perhaps the concern over possible immobilization of iron and other minerals by high dietary fibre has been overstated.

When the diet consists mainly of refined cereals (including white bread), sugar, and fats, the cereals then become the sole, if somewhat poor, source of iron. Such diets were studied in the poverty-stricken communities of Aberdeen during the depression of the 1930s, when the food eaten was dictated by economic factors rather than by choice. Daily intakes of iron were only of the order of 7.7mg, which is about half the desirable minimum. Fortification of white flour was unheard of at that time, so not surprisingly iron deficiency was prevalent in these communities. Even today diets consisting mainly of refined cereals are not uncommon in the Third World countries, and amongst certain population groups in the more affluent countries, such diets are eaten by choice.

Food processing can also increase the iron content, albeit unwittingly. For example, by the time fresh orange juice is canned, its action on the metal machinery can increase its iron concentration five-fold. At the same time, however, the tin content can increase some ten times because of the acidity of the juice. Commercial processing of foods in iron vessels or domestic cooking in iron pots can contribute extra iron to the food when eaten. In fact, in parts of Africa, communal cooking vessels can be dissolved to such an extent that toxic levels of iron are introduced into the food and the people eating it. Conversely, in industrial food processing replacement of cast-iron equipment with stainless steel has significantly reduced the iron contamination of some foods.

Milk is a poor source of iron, with human breast milk containing only slightly more than that from cows. Hence infants may be prone to iron deficiency because the iron content of cow's milk is low and the quantity of the mineral passed on by the mother during development until birth is usually not sufficient to meet the child's needs beyond the age of six months. By then mixed feeding has usually started and other foods can start contributing iron. Baby milk preparations made from dried cow's milk are usually fortified with iron to ensure adequate intake. This is not possible with human breast milk; in some poorer Third World communities it is not unusual for breast-feeding to continue for up to two years and both mother and child invariably suffer from iron deficiency.

Dietary sources

There is no doubt that the richest dietary sources of iron are foods of animal, poultry, and fish origin, which have the added advantage of containing the mineral in the haem form, the more efficiently absorbed type. Even amongst these foods, however, there are wide variations in iron content. Red meats tend to contain more iron than white meats and offal is richer than muscle meats. Pride of place goes to pig's and lamb's liver (21.0 and 9.4mg per 100g respectively), with kidney bringing up second place, lamb, ox, and pig respectively providing 7.4, 5.7, and 5.0mg per 100g. These are the figures for the raw meats. When fried the concentration of iron in these meats is even higher because of loss of water in the cooking process (see Table 2). Muscle meats in general provide between 1.9 and 3.5mg per 100g. Traditional black puddings and blood sausages are the richest sources of iron in meat and offal products (up to 29mg iron per 100g) because they are blood-based, and as the iron is haem iron, its availability to the body is excellent.

Table 2 Iron content of food items, products, and prepared dishes as eaten (mg per 100g food)

Meats

Beef steak	3.4	Pork leg	1.3
Beef joint	2.8	Pork chop	1.2
Beef mince	2.7	Bacon	1.5-1.6
Lamb leg	2.7	Veal cutlet	1.6
Lamb shoulder	1.8	Veal fillet	1.6
Lamb chop	2.1		

Poultry and game birds

Chicken light meat	0.5	Goose	4.6
Chicken dark meat	1.0	Grouse	7.6
Turkey light meat	0.5	Partridge	7.7
Turkey dark meat	1.4	Pheasant	8.4
Duck	2.7	Pigeon	19.4

Game

Hare	10.8
Rabbit	1.9
Venison	7.8

Offal

Brain	1.4-2.3	Liver calf	7.5
Heart sheep	8.1	Liver chicken	9.1
Heart ox	7.7	Liver lamb	10.0
Heart lamb	3.6	Liver ox	7.8
Kidney lamb	12.0	Liver pig	17.0
Kidney ox	8.0	Tongue sheep	3.4
Kidney pig	6.4	Tongue ox	4.9
Sweetbread	1.8	Tripe	0.7

Meat products

Corned beef	2.9	Sausages beef	1.7
Ham	1.2	Sausages pork	1.5
Luncheon meat	1.1	Beefburgers	3.1
Stewed steak	2.1	Meat paste	2.3
Black pudding	20.0	Steak and kidney pie	2.8
Haggis	4.8	Hot pot	1.2
Liver sausage	6.4	Irish stew	0.6
Frankfurters	1.5	Moussaka	1.3
Salami	1.0	Shepherd's pie	1.1

Meat dishes

Beef stew	0.7	Pork chow mein	0.7
Stuffed peppers	1.2	Beans and frankfurters	1.6
Chilli con carne	1.4	Ham quiche	0.6
Spaghetti with meat		Ham fritters	1.6
sauce	1.5		
Chicken pie	1.0		

White fish

Cod baked	0.4	Sole fried	1.1
Cod fried	0.5	Sole steamed	0.6
Cod grilled	0.4	Plaice fried batter	1.0
Cod poached	0.3	Plaice fried crumbs	0.8
Cod steamed	0.5	Plaice steamed	0.6
Haddock fried	1.2	Saithe steamed	0.6
Haddock steamed	0.7	Whiting fried	0.7
Haddock smoked	1.0	Whiting steamed	1.0
Halibut steamed	0.6		

Fatty fish

Eel stewed	0.9	Salmon stewed	0.8
Herring fried	1.0	Salmon canned	1.4
Herring grilled	1.0	Salmon smoked	0.6
Bloater grilled	2.2	Sardines canned in oil	2.9
Kipper baked	1.4	Sardines canned in	
Mackerel fried	1.2	tomato sauce	4.6
Pilchards canned	2.7	Sprats fried	4.0
Trout	1.0	Tuna canned	1.1
		Whitebait	5.1

Cartilaginous fish

Dogfish and skate	0.8-1.1

Crustacea

Crab boiled	1.3
Crab canned	2.8
Lobster boiled	0.8
Prawns boiled	1.1
Scampi fried	1.1
Shrimps boiled	1.8
Shrimps canned	5.1

Molluscs

Cockles boiled	26.0
Mussels boiled	7.7
Oysters raw	6.0
Scallops steams	3.0
Whelks boiled	6.2
Winkles boiled	15.0

Fish products and dishes

Fish cakes fried	1.0
Fish fingers fried	0.7
Fish paste	9.0
Fish pie	0.4
Kedgeree	0.9
Roe hard fried	1.6
Roe soft fried	1.5
Tuna casserole	1.1

Cereals and cereal products

Arrowroot	2.0	Spaghetti boiled	0.4
Barley boiled	0.2	Spaghetti canned	0.4
Wheatgerm	10.0	Tapioca pudding	0.03
Wheatbran	12.9	Bread wholemeal	2.5
Cornflour	1.4	Bread brown	2.5
Custard powder	1.4	Bread white	1.7
Flour wholemeal	4.0	All-Bran	12.0
Flour brown	3.6	Cornflakes	0.6
Flour white	2.2	Grapenuts	5.2
Macaroni boiled	0.5	Muesli	4.6
Oatmeal raw	4.1	Puffed Wheat	4.6
Porridge	0.5	Ready Brek	4.9
Rice white boiled	0.2	Rice Krispies	0.7
Rice brown boiled	1.0	Shredded Wheat	4.2
Rye flour	2.7	Special K	20.0
Sago pudding	0.2	Sugar Puffs	2.1
Semolina pudding	0.1	Weetabix	7.6
Sago flour full fat	6.9	Crispbread	3.7-5.4
Sago flour low fat	9.1	Cream crackers	1.7

Flour Products

Biscuits chocolate	1.7	Cakes fancy	1.4
Biscuits digestive	2.0	Cakes fruit	1.8
Biscuits ginger	4.0	Cakes gingerbread	3.8
Biscuits oatcakes	4.5	Cakes Madeira	1.1
Biscuits sandwich	1.6	Cakes rock	1.4
Biscuits semi-sweet	2.1	Cakes sponge	1.4
Biscuits short-sweet	1.8	Cakes sponge and jam	1.6
Biscuits shortbread	1.5	Buns	2.5
Biscuits wafer filled	1.6	Doughnuts	1.9
Biscuits wafer	1.6	Tarts jam	1.6
Scones	1.5	Tarts mince	1.7
Scotch pancakes	1.3	Pastry	1.5-1.8

Puddings

Apple crumble	0.6	Meringues	0.1
Bread and butter pudding	0.7	Milk pudding	0.1
Cheesecake	0.7	Milk pudding canned	0.2
Christmas pudding	1.9	Pancakes	0.9
Egg custard	0.5	Sponge pudding	1.2
Custard tart	1.0	Suet pudding	0.9
Dumplings	0.8	Treacle tart	1.5
Fruit pie	0.6-1.2	Trifle	0.7
Ice-cream	0.2-0.3	Yorkshire pudding	1.0
Jelly water	0.4		
Jelly milk	0.4		
Lemon meringue pie	1.0		

Milk and milk products

Milk, fresh, whole	0.03-0.06	Cheese Camembert	0.76
Milk sterilized	0.05	Cheese Cheddar	0.40
Milk UHT	0.05	Cheese Danish blue	0.17
Milk fresh, skimmed	0.05	Cheese Edam	0.21
Milk condensed	0.20	Cheese Parmesan	0.37
Milk condensed,		Cheese Stilton	0.46
skimmed	0.29	Cheese cottage	0.10
Milk evaporated	0.20	Cheese cream	0.12
Milk dried whole	0.40	Cheese processed	0.50
Milk dried, skimmed	0.40	Cheese spread	0.69
Milk human	0.07	Yogurt natural	0.09
Milk colostrum	0.07	Yogurt flavoured	0.16
Butter	0.16	Yogurt fruit	0.24

Cream single	0.31	Yogurt nut	0.23
Cream double	0.20		
Cream whipping	0.25		
Cream canned	0.30		

Eggs		**Egg/cheese dishes**	
Whole raw	2.0	Cauliflower cheese	0.4
White raw	0.1	Cheese pudding	0.8
Yolk raw	6.1	Cheese soufflé	1.1
Dried	7.9	Macaroni cheese	0.4
Boiled	2.0	Pizza	1.1
Fried	2.5	Quiche	1.3
Poached	2.3	Scotch egg	1.7
Omelette	1.7	Welsh rabbit	1.1
Scrambled	1.7		

Oils and fats all contain between 0 and 0.4mg iron per 100g.

Vegetables

RICH SOURCES, greater than 2.5mg per 100g as eaten.

Haricot beans	2.5	Mung beans	2.6
Red kidney beans	6.2	Endive raw	2.8
Laverbread	3.5	Split lentils	2.5
Parsley	8.0	Bengal peas dahl	3.1
Spinach boiled	4.0	Turnip tops boiled	3.1

GOOD SOURCES, between 1.0 and 2.4mg per 100g as eaten.

Broad beans	1.0	Peas boiled	1.2
Butter beans	1.7	Peas frozen boiled	1.4
Baked beans	1.4	Peas canned garden	1.5
Beansprouts canned	1.0	Peas canned processed	1.6
Broccoli tops boiled	1.0	Peas dried boiled	1.4
Carrots canned	1.3	Peas split boiled	1.7
Horseradish	2.0	Bengal channa dahl	1.8
Leeks	2.0	Chipped potatoes frozen	1.0
Masur dahl	1.7	Potato powder	2.4
Mushrooms raw	1.0	Potato crisps	2.1
Mushrooms fried	1.3	Radishes	1.9
Mustard and cress	1.0	Salsify	1.2
Okra	1.0	Spring greens	1.3
Spring onions	1.2	Watercress	1.6

MODERATE SOURCES, up to 1.0mg per 100g as eaten.

Achee canned	0.7	Cucumber	0.3
Artichokes	0.2–0.5	Lettuce	0.9
Asparagus	0.5	Marrow boiled	0.2
Aubergine raw	0.4	Onions raw	0.3
Beans French	0.6	Onions boiled	0.3
Beans runner	0.7	Onions fried	0.6
Beetroot	0.4	Parsnips	0.5
Brussels sprouts	0.5	Peppers raw	0.4
Cabbage red	0.6	Peppers boiled	0.4
Cabbage savoy	0.7	Plantain raw	0.5
Cabbage spring	0.5	Plantain boiled	0.4
Cabbage white	0.4	Plantain fried	0.8
Cabbage winter	0.4	Potatoes boiled	0.3
Carrots old raw	0.6	Potatoes mashed	0.3
Carrots old boiled	0.4	Potatoes baked	0.8
Carrots young boiled	0.4	Potatoes roast	0.7
Carrots young canned	1.3	Potatoes chipped	0.9
Cauliflower raw	0.5	Potatoes instant mashed	0.5
Cauliflower boiled	0.4	Pumpkin	0.4
Celeriac	0.8	Seakale	0.6
Celery raw	0.6	Swedes	0.3
Celery boiled	0.4	Sweetcorn	0.9
Chicory	0.7	Sweet potatoes	0.6
Tomatoes raw	0.4	Turnips	0.4
Tomatoes fried	0.5	Yam	0.3
Tomatoes canned	0.9		

Fruit

RICH SOURCES, 2.5mg or more per 100g as eaten.

Dried apricots raw	4.1
Dried figs, green raw	4.2
Dried peaches raw	6.8
Dried peaches stewed	2.5
Dried prunes raw	2.9

GOOD SOURCES, between 1.0 and 2.4mg per 100g as eaten.

Stewed apricots	1.5	Loganberries raw	1.4
Avocado pears	1.5	Loganberries stewed	1.3
Cranberries raw	1.1	Loganberries canned	1.4

Blackcurrants raw	1.3	Mulberries raw	1.6
Blackcurrants stewed	1.1	Olives in brine	1.0
Redcurrants raw	1.2	Passion fruit raw	1.1
Redcurrants stewed	1.0	Prunes stewed	1.4
Dried currants	1.8	Dried raisins	1.6
Dried dates	1.6	Raspberries raw	1.2
Figs stewed	2.3	Raspberries stewed	1.2
Fruit salad canned	1.0	Raspberries canned	1.7
Sultanas dried	1.8		

MODERATE SOURCES, up to 0.9mg per 100g as eaten.

Apricots canned	0.7	Mandarins canned	0.4
Bananas raw	0.4	Mangoes raw	0.5
Bilberries raw	0.7	Mangoes canned	0.4
Blackberries raw	0.9	Melons cantaloupe	0.8
Blackberries stewed	0.8	Melons honeydew	0.2
Cherries raw	0.4	Melons water	0.3
Whitecurrants raw	0.9	Nectarines raw	0.5
Whitecurrants stewed	0.8	Oranges raw	0.3
Damsons raw	0.4	Orange juice	0.3
Damons stewed	0.3	Pawpaw canned	0.4
Figs green raw	0.4	Peaches fresh raw	0.4
Fruit pie filling canned	0.5	Peaches canned	0.4
Gooseberries green raw	0.3	Pears eating	0.2
Gooseberries stewed	0.3	Pears cooking	0.2
Gooseberries ripe raw	0.6	Pears canned	0.3
Grapes, red and white	0.3	Pineapple fresh	0.4
Grapefruit raw	0.3	Pineapple canned	0.4
Grapefruit canned	0.7	Pineapple juice	0.7
Grapefruit juice	0.3	Plums Victoria	0.4
Greengages raw	0.4	Plums stewed	0.3
Greengages stewed	0.4	Pomegranate juice	0.2
Guavas canned	0.5	Quinces raw	0.3
Lemons whole	0.4	Rhubarb stewed	0.4
Lemon juice	0.1	Strawberries raw	0.7
Lychees raw	0.5	Strawberries canned	0.9
Lychees canned	0.7	Tangerines raw	0.3
Tomato juice	0.5		

Nuts
All are good or rich sources of iron as eaten.

Almonds	4.2	Coconut fresh	2.1
Barcelona nuts	3.0	Coconut desiccated	3.6
Brazils	2.8	Coconut milk	0.1
Chestnuts	0.9	Peanuts fresh or roasted	2.0
Cob or hazel	1.1	Peanut butter	2.1
Walnuts	2.4		

Other foods (including confectionery)

Sugar demerara	0.9	Boiled sweets	0.4
Sugar raw cane	5.0	Chocolate milk	1.6
Syrup golden	1.5	Chocolate plain	2.4
Treacle black	9.2	Chocolate filled	1.8
Molasses	8.0	Fruit gums	4.2
Honey	0.4	Liquorice sweets	8.1
Jam	1.0–1.5	Pastilles	1.4
Lemon curd	0.6	Peppermint	0.2
Marmalade	0.6	Toffee	1.5
Marzipan	2.0	Mincemeat	1.5

Beverages (including alcoholic drinks)

Cocoa powder	10.5	All beers and lagers	0.01–0.05
Coffee ground	4.1	Cider	0.5
Coffee infused	Trace	Wine red	0.9
Coffee instant	4.4	Wine rosé	1.0
Drinking chocolate	2.4	Wine white	0.5–1.21
Tea dried leaves	15.2	Port	0.4
Tea infused	Trace	Sherry	0.37–0.53
		Vermouth	0.35

Sauces and spices

Brown sauce	3.1	Bovril	14.0
Chutney	1.0	Curry powder	75–95
Mayonnaise	0.7	Ginger ground	17.2
Piccalilli	0.9	Marmite	3.7
Pickle sweet	2.0	Oxo cubes	24.5
Salad cream	0.8	Mustard powder	10.9
Tomato ketchup	1.2	Pepper	10.2
Tomato purée	5.1	Vinegar	0.5
Tomato sauce	0.3	Yeast compressed	5.0
		Yeast dried	20.0

Soups, as served, provide between 0.4 and 1.2mg per 100g.

Fish are useful providers of iron, but the white variety (range 0.6 to 1.1mg per 100g) is inferior to the fatty kind (range 0.7 to 4.6mg per 100g). Shellfish are divided into crustacea (e.g. crab, lobster, prawns, scampi), which contain between 0.3 and 1.8mg per 100g, and molluscs (e.g. mussels, oysters, scallops, winkles, and whelks), which are some ten times richer in iron (range 3.0 to 20mg per 100g). Cockles are the richest source of iron with an average content of 26.0mg, although levels of 40mg per 100g have been recorded.

As with meats, the darker flesh of poultry is richer in iron than is the white flesh (1.9 and 0.5mg per 100g respectively). Water birds like duck contain much higher quantities of the mineral, but the richest source of it amongst birds is game. Grouse and partridge provide an average of 7.6mg per 100g, but roast pigeon is by far the richest in providing 19.4mg iron per 100g. It is not certain why such high concentrations of the mineral are present in game birds, but it could reflect a free-range diet. A similar situation is seen in animal game (e.g. hare, rabbit, venison), which contain higher amounts of iron than domesticated animals, so here too the reason may be the free-range and varied diet.

Vegetarians and vegans

Those who confine themselves to eating plant foods and in some cases dairy products are deprived of the haem iron present in foods of animal, fish, and poultry origin, so the whole of their dietary iron is of the non-haem type. This means that the bioavailability of the mineral is less, but what these diets lack in quality they make up for in quantity. As dairy products are essentially poor sources of iron both vegetarians and vegans (extreme vegetarians who partake of no foods of animal, fish, or poultry origin) obtain their iron from similar items of foods. Despite this, there is no evidence that either group are any more iron deficient than meat eaters.

A study reported in the *Proceedings of the Nutrition Society* in 1967 indicated that, in general, iron intakes of vegans tended to be greater than those of omnivores (meat-eaters). The same study looked at the incidence of iron-deficiency anaemia in both vegans and omnivores and found no difference. In another study reported in the *American Journal of Clinical Nutrition* in 1984, iron intakes of omnivores were compared to those of lactovegetarians (i.e. eggs, milk, and dairy products form part of their diet) and vegans. Again in all cases, iron intakes satisfied current requirements and in no case did clinical and biochemical investigation of the subjects reveal any signs of nutritional deficiency.

Unrefined wholegrains, oatmeal, brown rice, and various flours are good sources of iron (between 1.0 and 4.1mg per 100g). Soya products and the low-fat soya flour in particular supply even more iron (up to 9.1mg per 100g), placing them on a par with meat products, except of course that the iron in these plant foods is not assimilated as well as that from meats. Molasses is an extremely rich source because the product is what is left from raw cane sugar after all the sucrose (sugar) has been removed. Since raw cane sugar (unlike the white variety) contains more than one milligram of iron per 100g, this can be concentrated a hundred times as the white sugar, which is devoid of iron, is crystallized out and removed.

Vegetables are all good sources of iron, with concentrated foods like pulses (peas, beans and lentils) extremely rich in the mineral with levels of up to 8.0mg per 100g. Although green-leafed vegetables are lower in concentration of iron than other vegetables they do contain higher potencies of vitamin C. As we shall see later this vitamin can enhance the absorption of iron derived from plants, so the mineral from green-leafed vegetables (low iron, high vitamin C) is used just as efficiently as that from other vegetables (high iron, low vitamin C).

Fresh fruits all contain some iron (up to 0.5mg per 100g), but the vitamin C present will ensure it is absorbed efficiently. Dried fruits, on the other hand, contain more than ten times the iron of their fresh counterparts but they are virtually devoid of vitamin C, which is lost during the drying process. The end result of eating both types of fruit is a similar uptake of iron during the absorption process because of this variation in vitamin C content. Dried apricots, for example, supply 4.1mg of iron per 100g compared to only 0.4mg in the fresh, raw fruit.

Nature is generous in her provision of iron across the whole range of foodstuffs. No one who is conscious of their diet need suffer from iron deficiency in their intakes. Vegetarians and vegans are usually more aware and careful of what they eat than are omnivores, which is why they suffer no more iron deficiency than anyone else. One word of warning, however. Sometimes one vegetarian in a family of omnivores may simply be fed conventional meals minus the meat. This practice can lead to problems if the lack of meat is not compensated for by increased intakes of vegetables and other non-meat sources of iron.

The iron contents of various food items, food products, and prepared food dishes are shown in Table 2. All figures are in mg iron per 100g food (approximately 3.5 ounces), in many cases an average portion. The amounts of iron can vary when in the same foodstuffs and the quantities tabulated are the average of a number of estimations.

Iron, as well as being derived from constituents occurring naturally in foods, may also be contributed by metallic contamination either from processing machinery, kitchen knives, pots and pans, or from particles of soil, especially in vegetables. This contamination of foods from one source or another is probably a major source of variation, but even so, wide ranges of values are often reported in the literature under circumstances where precautions had been taken to avoid contamination. Such figures probably represent soil variation.

In addition, iron compounds are added to a number of important foods, and these augmented figures will appear in the table. There is statutory addition of iron in the UK and in many other countries to all wheat flours except wholemeal. Many proprietary breakfast cereals and baby foods contain added iron, mainly to replace that lost during the refining of the naturally occurring food.

————Where we get our dietary iron————

The figures in Table 2 illustrate how widely iron is distributed in the foods we eat, and with such a large spread it is difficult to imagine anyone not receiving sufficient in the diet. Nevertheless in the UK, the Ministry of Agriculture, Fisheries, and Food (MAFF) evaluate the intakes of iron from various food items each year in various households, and indeed have done so for the past 100 years or so. Two methods have been used to estimate the national average intakes of iron and other trace minerals.

The first is based on MAFF's National Food Survey, which is

a continuous survey of 7,500 households selected at random throughout Britain each year. The individual responsible for buying food records the type, amount, and cost of each item brought into the home. Alcoholic drinks and sweets are disregarded because the information on them is liable to be inaccurate. Meals and snacks eaten outside the home are also excluded because of the difficulties encountered in obtaining accurate descriptions and in assessing quantities of foods eaten by all family members, particularly children.

Take-away meals, picnics, and lunches made from food items bought for the household food supply are assessed since they can be evaluated in the home. The amounts of each food and their cost are noted each week and the information is supplied to the Ministry. Here the basic nutritional value of the diets can be calculated and all the data is published annually by HMSO under the general title Ministry of Agriculture, Fisheries, and Food, *Household Food Consumption and Expenditure* (annual reports of the National Food Survey Committee). The figures allow the intakes of foods and hence the nutrients in those foods (including iron) to be assessed per household, and average amounts per individual in that household can also be worked out.

The second way of estimating national average intakes of iron and other micronutrients has been via the chemical analysis of food samples from the 'total diet study'. This is based on assessing the iron content of 68 key foods (the amounts are based on the National Food Survey information but with the inclusion of sweets, water, and soft drinks) which were bought at intervals by colleges specializing in home economics, departments of food science or similar organizations. The foods were prepared and cooked where appropriate, grouped, and then analysed for their iron content at the Laboratory of the Government Chemist (LGC).

In addition, MAFF and LGC have analysed a wide variety of individual food items from among the five to ten thousand foods available in the UK. In fact most of the proportions of iron quoted in Table 2 have been taken from figures published by MAFF as the fourth revised and extended edition of Medical Research Council Special Report No. 297, known more familiarly as McCance and Widdowson's, *The Composition of Foods*, ed. A. A. Paul and D. A. T. Southgate (HMSO, 1978).

The foods assessed were chosen because they are important in the nation's diet as a whole for particular groups (e.g. bread, milk, potatoes, breakfast cereals, infant foods, alcoholic drink) or because evidence from other countries suggested that they would be particularly rich in iron and other trace minerals (e.g. offal and shellfish). The samples in the studies were as representative of the food items eaten in Britain as possible. They were bought at a variety of retail outlets, often at different times of the year, and particular care was taken to ensure that all major brands of processed foods were assayed for micronutrient content.

There is also a third way of measuring how much of each nutrient and micronutrient we are actually eating, and because this technique is used on individuals it is the best method for assessing a person's actual intake. The subject notes down in a diary the exact amount of each food item they eat at every meal for a week. Ideally the items are weighed, but whilst this is easily carried out when at home, it is recognized that when eating out amounts must be assessed. Any food not eaten is also weighed, so the exact amount eaten is known. At the end of the week, the completed diaries are taken to a nutritionist who is able to work out individual nutrient and micronutrient values for each food item from standard tables such as those in *The Composition of Foods* published by McCance and Widdowson's. Hence it is possible to know how much iron, for example, was contributed by each food item and, of course, iron intakes per meal, per day, or per week. This is a well-established method and was the one used in the study reported in the Booker Health Report I that was carried out on 801 individuals from 449 households. The results indicated that 60 per cent of women in the 18–54 age range have iron intakes below the Recommended Daily Amount.

When the amounts of iron we eat are calculated from the National Food Survey and compared to those calculated from the Total Diet Study, the figures are in reasonable agreement. During the ten years or so both have been in existence, comparisons have been good. The advantage of both methods, of course, is that trends in what we are eating can be assessed and possible changes in the make-up of our diets and the contributions of various foodstuffs to nutrient intakes are revealed.

Table 3 compares the average total dietary iron intakes of

individuals using the two methods. Table 4 goes further in that the contribution of the major groups of foods to iron intakes is compared in both methods. Table 5 shows how the way in which various foodstuffs contribute to our iron intake has changed between 1973 and 1981.

Table 3 Comparison of two methods for estimating national average intakes of iron

National average intakes of iron (mg per person per day)

Year	National Food Survey	Total Diet Study (± standard deviation)
1976	11.5	13.4 ± 3.5
1977	11.0	12.2 ± 1.7
1978	11.2	11.7 ± 2.2
1979	11.0	
1980	11.3	11.9 ± 1.9
1981	10.9	11.2 ± 1.5

Table 4 Contributions of major groups of food to iron intakes for 1981

Foodstuff	National Food Survey		Total Diet Study	
	mg/day	per cent	mg/day	per cent
Cereals	4.1	37	5.1	45
Meat and eggs	3.1	29	2.8	25
Fish	0.2	2	0.2	2
Milk	0.2	2	0.4	4
Fats and other dairy products	0.2	2	0.1	1
Root vegetables	0.8	7	0.8	7
Other vegetables	1.1	11	0.9	8
Fruits and sugar products	0.6	5	0.7	6
Beverages	0.1	1	0.2	2
Other foods	0.5	4	—	—

It can be seen from Tables 4 and 5 that absolute levels of iron, trends in intake since 1976, and contributions made to the total by most of the major food groups are all in reasonable agreement. Cereals are an exception: in 1981 their contribution to iron intake was higher in the Total Diet Study. However, in 1980 agreement was better. The figures were 4.4mg (39 per cent of the total) and 4.5mg (38 per cent of the total) respectively for the National Food Survey and Total Diet Study.

Some differences might be expected between the two methods of study since the inclusion of chocolate, sugar confectionary, and soft drinks in the Total Diet Study would tend to increase the value of the iron intake as chocolate is a good source of the mineral. On the other hand, meat, vegetables, and fish are cooked before being eaten and there could therefore be some loss of iron into the cooking water.

Table 5 Changes in dietary sources of iron between 1973 and 1981

Foodstuffs	1973 mg iron per day	1981 mg iron per day
Cereals (including bread)	4.0	4.1
Meat and eggs	4.2	3.1
Fish	0.2	0.2
Milk, fats, and dairy products	0.7	0.4
Root vegetables	1.0	0.8
Other vegetables	1.5	1.1
Fruit and sugar	0.5	0.6
Beverages	0.2	0.1
Other foods		0.5
	12.3	10.9

All figures are taken from the National Food Survey for those years. The reduction in iron intake in 1981 is significant and the main reason appears to be a decrease in iron derived from meat and eggs, dairy products, and vegetables other than root. One worrying aspect is the significant loss of iron by a reduction in meat products eaten. Eggs are insignificant providers of iron because of the poor availability of the mineral, so the decrease in meat intake provides the main reason for the shortfall. As meat also supplies iron in the best-absorbed form, the overall result is that less iron is available to the individual. In addition, it looks as if the iron lost by eating less or no meat is not being made up elsewhere.

The apparent reduced intake of dairy products and milk in 1981 compared to 1973 probably reflects the increased concern of the public concerning eating saturated fats and cholesterol between the two surveys. Less iron is also being obtained from non-root vegetables, and the decreased intake of these foodstuffs can also have other consequences such as lower dietary levels of vitamin C, folic acid, and dietary fibre. As we shall see later, all of these are associated with iron in its metabolic and nutritional roles.

One advantage of the National Food Survey approach is that it allows contributions from individual foods as well as from food groups to be estimated. It indicated for example that of the 11mg of iron in the diet in 1977, 1.1mg was derived from food fortification (largely from statutory additions to white and brown flour); 1.3mg was haem iron (from meat, fish, and poultry); and the remaining 8.6mg was non-haem iron (from fruit, cereals, vegetables, and nuts). The study also showed that food intakes provided between 98 and 105 per cent of the UK Recommended Daily Amount of iron between 1976 and 1981 after allowing for the proportion of meals not taken from the domestic food supply and for wastage.

─────Iron fortification of foods and drinks─────

Addition of iron to white and brown (but not wholemeal) flour has been mandatory in the UK since 1953 to replace losses of the mineral during milling. Although the added iron was never intended as a means of preventing or treating iron-deficiency anaemia, nutrient needs and food choices of specific population groups (e.g. young children, adolescents, and women of child-bearing age), the development of diabetic and low-energy products, the overall trend towards consuming fewer calories, and the greater reliance on snack foods are just some of the reasons why food fortification is still regarded as necessary. At the same time, advances in food technology and new manufacturing processes have created opportunities to add iron to foods and drinks. Replacement of meats with soya protein products has also raised questions about iron availability from both types of food since the mineral in meats is far better absorbed. Fortification is one way to ensure that soya protein products provide enough iron to give the same sort of bioavailability as meat iron to the person eating them.

Bioavailability is the amount of iron actually absorbed into the body from different meals. It is not a simple sum of the absorption of the iron from the single foods contained in that meal. It is the net effect of the amounts and properties of the iron compounds present in all food items and of all the factors present that can increase or decrease iron absorption. It is for these reasons that recent studies on iron absorption have measured it from meals rather than from individual food items. Most of these studies have come from Professor L. Hallberg of the Department of Medicine, University of Göteborg, Sweden, and some of his published results are shown in Tables 10, 11, and 12 (see pages 79, 80, and 81 respectively). These results are highly significant because as they are taken from meals as eaten, they are more meaningful in determining just how much iron we eat is actually assimilated.

The main criteria for selecting types of iron that may be added to foods are that they are necessary, safe, and effective. Addition of iron is accomplished using the techniques of restoration and fortification, both of which are often described as enrichment. Strictly speaking, restoration refers to replacement of nutrients where losses cannot be avoided during handling, processing, and storage of foods, and a good example is iron depletion during the refining of wholemeal flour. By the same token, fortification refers to addition of nutrients that were not present in the original food (e.g. vitamins A and D added to margarine) but can apply equally well to addition of nutrients that were present in the food but only in nutritionally insignificant amounts. To some nutritionists this also applies to white flour.

There is no doubt that nutrient enrichment of foods can help prevent nutritional inadequacies in a population where there is a risk of deficiency or when intervention is needed to correct a proven deficiency in an identified sector of the population. A prime example is Sweden, where the iron added to flour and other foods contributes 35 per cent of the total iron dietary intake. The result is a marked drop in the prevalence of iron deficiency in that country in women of child-bearing age during the past 15 years or so. It has been calculated that iron fortification of flour can account for about one-third of this reduction in anaemia. Other factors include the use of oral contraceptives, which reduce menstrual losses of iron by half, and the increasing tendency to take iron supplements and vitamin C.

Ultimately, the criterion of effectiveness of iron fortification is whether or not nutrition status and health have been improved. Nutrition additions can also be part of a marketing and promotional strategy, e.g. in cereals, where there is no mandatory fortification but extra iron helps sell more of the product. Nutrient content can be a significant factor in establishing a market for a particular product such as prepared breakfast cereals. Research has shown that when consumers compare products with a similar price, they favour those with more nutrients and those which have the longer list of nutrients on the label. In recent times this philosophy has been tempered somewhat by the attitude that long lists of ingredients are acceptable as long as they are not numbers prefixed by an 'E'. Nevertheless, the same research indicated that consumers are more willing to pay higher prices for foods fortified with nutrients if those products are regarded as nutritious, such as milk products and breakfast cereals, but not in snack foods and soft drinks. In the USA, the Food and Drug Administration has published guide-lines which discourage the indiscriminate additions of nutrients to foods.

Whilst we think mainly of the benefits of iron added to bread and cereal products in terms of ensuring adequate intakes, the mineral has also been added to several other components of the diet including table salt, monosodium glutamate, sugar, coffee, tea, oils, and fats. No matter to which food the iron is added, however, the benefits derived depend on the form of the iron salts employed, the uniformity of the food, and the composition of the meal and total diet in which the food item is eaten. In general, iron compounds that exhibit the best bioavailability in the person eating them also tend to have a higher chance of causing unwelcome effects in the food to which they are added. These can include undesirable colour, discernible taste, and a reduction in the shelf-life of the food. All may hinder consumer acceptability.

—Iron salts used as food sources of the mineral—

The major chemical characteristics of iron sources that determine their behaviour in foods are:

(i)   Their solubility. Ferrous iron salts are more soluble than ferric iron salts and so are more likely to be absorbed from the intestine.

(ii) Their state of oxidation. Ferrous iron salts (the lower state of oxidation) are more efficiently assimilated than ferric iron salts (the higher state of oxidation). However, ferrous salts tend to be reactive to the foods to which they are added.

(iii) Their ability to form complexes that are not available for assimilation. In general, ferric iron salts have a greater tendency to form these complexes.

According to the Bread and Flour Regulations 1984 Schedule 1, iron must be added to white and brown flour at a level of not less than 1.65mg per 100g flour. In addition, the same schedule specifies the forms of iron salts, either singly or in combination, that may be used to fortify the flour. They are ferric ammonium citrate, ferrous sulphate BP, dried ferrous sulphate BP, and iron powder. The purity of the two forms of ferric ammonium citrate are specified in another part of the Food Regulations; both types of ferrous sulphate must be of the standard laid down in the British Pharmacopoeia. Iron powder is defined as consisting essentially

Table 6 Some iron sources in current use for fortification

Iron Compound	Other common names	Iron content (%)	RBV
Ferric phosphate	Ferric orthophosphate	28	3–46
Ferric pyrophosphate	Iron pyrophosphate	25	45
Ferric sodium Pyrophosphate	Sodium iron Pyrophosphate	15	14
Ferric ammonium Citrate	Green ferric ammonium Citrate	17	107
Ferrous fumarate		33	95
Ferrous gluconate		12	97
Ferrous lactate		38	—
Ferrous sulphate	Dried ferrous sulphate	32	100
Iron powder	Elemental iron Ferrum reductum Metallic iron	100	—
Reduced iron (hydrogen process)		96	34
Reduced iron (electrolytic process)		97	50
Reduced iron (carbonyl process)		98	67

of finely divided metallic iron containing not less than 90 per cent by weight of iron. It is a fine greyish-black powder of specified particle size.

These iron sources are confined to flour, but additional iron salts may be added to other foods both here in the UK and elsewhere in the world. The most commonly used are shown in Table 6. The Relative Biological Value (RBV) refers to the efficiency of the iron preparation in curing deficiency in rats compared to ferrous sulphate. The criteria for determining cure are the blood haemoglobin content and the haematocrit level (i.e. the volume of red blood cells packed into a given volume of blood).

Iron fortification of flour

Many studies have cast doubt on the effectiveness of adding iron to flour because of queries regarding just how much of the added iron is actually absorbed. One report, by Dr P. C. Elwood of the Medical Research Council Epidemiological Research Unit, Cardiff, was entitled 'Radio-active studies of the absorption by human subjects of various iron preparations from bread'. This study compared two labelled forms of iron powder with radioactive labelled ferric ammonium sulphate and ferrous sulphate (both salts approved for flour) in regard to their absorption from single meals. Radioactive labelled iron salts are often used in absorption experiments because the body cannot distinguish this 'marked' iron from iron in foods, and because the radioactive material is easily detected and measured, its uptake is readily calculated. The results indicated that more of the iron in the two iron salts was absorbed than from the iron powder.

In a second study, reported in *The Lancet* in 1968, Dr Elwood reports results of a community feeding trial lasting nine months and involving 237 anaemic women. The haemoglobin levels of the blood of these women were measured after feeding them bread fortified with either ferric ammonium citrate or with ferrous sulphate. Very little benefit on the haemoglobin levels was observed with ferric ammonium citrate compared to ferrous sulphate.

Powdered electrolytically precipitated iron is scarcely absorbed at all and there is little if any therapeutic benefit from ferric ammonium citrate, so Elwood in *Clinical Science* in 1971 concludes that iron added to flour used to bake bread is very poorly available to man in a normal diet. The conclusion was confirmed in another study in the USA by Drs S. T. Callender and G. T. Warner, who reported in the *American Journal of Nutrition* (1968). They went further, however, and showed enhanced absorption of iron with bread when given with orange juice, presumably because of the latter's vitamin C content.

The poor absorption of iron from flour cannot be compensated for by adding more iron, since iron salts induce rancidity on storing and adversely affect baking quantities. From several years' work on the effect of adding iron to flour in the UK the sad conclusion emerges that these supplements are of little value to the population. It is because of these negative results that in 1980 the Committee on Medical Aspects of Food Policy in their DHSS Report on Health and Social Subjects, 23, 'Nutritional Aspects of Bread and Flour', Report of the Panel on Bread, Flour, and other Cereal Products (HMSO, 1981), pp. 1–64, decided that there was no nutritional advantage in continued compulsory addition of iron to flour. However, at the time of writing iron fortification of flour is still mandatory under the Bread and Flour Regulations 1984.

There is a postscript to the 1981 report mentioned above. According to researchers at the Institute of Food Research at Norwich, reduced iron powder may not be as useless as the 1981 report suggests. They suggest that the particle size of the reduced iron added to flour is a critical factor in determining the availability of the mineral. If the particles are above a certain size then absorption is virtually nil, but if they are below this size absorption is increased dramatically (see Table 6). The current regulations stipulate that 95 per cent of the particles in fortification iron should be less than the critical size of $50\mu m$ (micrometres). This means that the iron currently added to breads is probably significantly more available than the earlier studies would imply (*British Medical Journal* [12 July 1986], 139). Research to confirm this is currently being undertaken.

——Iron fortification of foods other than flour——

The ferric form of iron and its reduced ferrous form are the only states of the mineral that occur naturally in foods. Elemental iron is found rarely in biological systems, though it is used widely as an added nutrient. As the free metal iron is unlikely to react with other components of food it is used as a fortifying agent, but as we have seen, its availabilty is poor. Hence ferrous and ferric salts are more popular because of their better absorption, but they are more likely to react with other food ingredients.

Iron salts can (i) speed up vitamin degradation, particularly of vitamin C, thiamine (vitamin B1), and retinol (vitamin A) and so cause loss of nutritional value of a food. Ferric salts (but *not* ferrous) can also destroy vitamin E, so this too would be taken into account when deciding on a suitable fortifying agent. Ferric salts (ii) increase the speed and extent of rancidity of fats and oils. Iron salts act as catalysts in the reaction between atmospheric oxygen, and these nutrients (iii) produce undesirable colours, colour fading, off-flavours and undesirable precipitates, according to a report in the *British Journal of Nutrition* (1978).

Many of these effects occur as a result of interactions between the iron salts and naturally occurring food components such as anthocyanins (colouring agents), bioflavonoids, and tannins. For example, all iron salts will discolour dehydrated washed potato; a black colour results from interaction between ferrous salts and tannins in cocoa products; 'beer haze' is a term used to describe turbidity caused by reactions between iron, copper, tin, and calcium with the tannins and protein of beer.

In attempting to fortify foods with iron, it soon becomes evident that colour, texture, flavour, and quality control problems are greater for iron than for any other added nutrient. Such problems increase with greater concentrations of iron or as the serving size to include the desired iron addition is reduced. Including, say, 6mg of iron in a helping of cereal is easier than putting the same amount in a smaller quantity of a concentrated food. In addition, bioavailability and reactivity of iron sources may change during processing and storage of the food because of changes in the form of the iron. Extensive research is therefore necessary to determine the effect of a particular type of iron supplement on the food's composition and manufacture. Only then can evaluation of the fortifying agent be determined properly.

Although the ideal form of iron in theory is ferrous, this is readily converted to the less desirable ferric by other components of food or even the manufacturing process. Conversely, even when present in the ferric state, iron can be reduced to ferrous by natural food constituents like vitamin C. When this vitamin is present, as for example in fortified beverages, virtually all the iron is retained in the desirable ferrous form. Ferric salts, like ferric orthophosphate, under the influence of vitamin C become solubilized and converted to ferrous orthophosphate, when they are more readily accepted by the body. Whilst vitamin C is present, you may assume that any iron present is of the desired ferrous form. Vitamin C forms a combination product with ferrous iron called ferrous-ascorbic chelate, which is more stable than the ferric-ascorbic chelate complex between ferric iron and the vitamin. This vitamin is a factor in determining that ferrous iron is retained in that state in the fortified food.

Therefore the state of iron can change during processing and storage of the fortified food and it is also influenced by pH (acidity or alkalinity), presence of water, high temperature, and the content of other food constituents including those that are capable of chelating or 'complexing' the mineral. To these must be added the bioavailability, particle size, surface area, and purity of the iron source in order to ensure that whatever is being used to fortify the food can actually be absorbed by the body.

————Iron nutrition and fortification————

Despite apparent overwhelming evidence pointing to iron deficiency in many diets, the desirability of fortifying foods with iron is by no means generally accepted. Studies aiming to evaluate the effect of iron fortification nutritional status are sparse and generally deal with vegetable foods, in which the iron appears to be of low availability. Professor L. Hallberg, a leading Swedish researcher in iron metabolism, has questioned the practical value of iron fortification and has even considered it to be potentially harmful (*Seminars in Haematology* [1982]).

In the UK it is estimated that between 10 and 15 per cent of total iron intake is derived from food fortification; in the USA the amount has been suggested to be 25 per cent. A comprehensive study reported from Sweden (L. Hallberg *et al.* in *Bulletin of the World Health Organization* [1979]), where iron fortification accounts for 35 per cent of the iron intake, has indicated a striking fall in the prevalence of iron-deficiency anaemia from 25–30 per cent in the mid 1960s to 6–7 per cent between 1970 and 1980. After the first population studies the iron supplementation of flour was increased from 30mg per kg to 50mg per kg and extended to all types of flour. A further increase to 65mg per kg occurred in 1970. There were no major changes in dietary habits during this time and in 1973 50 per cent of the total dietary intake of iron resulted from fortification. This was shown to be effectively absorbed, and is calculated to account for a drop of 7–8 per cent in the prevalence of anaemia.

In addition to this source of extra iron, there was a remarkable change in Swedish habits during this period which resulted in a rise in consumption of iron tablets. In 1974 sales of iron in supplement form reached 5.8mg per day per head in Sweden, compared to only 1.0mg per day per head in the UK in the same year. The proportion of women of child-bearing age taking iron in Sweden rose from 16.9 per cent in 1963–4 to 27.5 per cent in 1974–5. To the increased voluntary iron intake must be added an increased intake of vitamin C, so this too contributed to the reduced incidence of non-iron-deficiency anaemia. Despite world-wide controversy over the value of iron fortification of foods, the Swedish experience does indicate that positive benefits can be derived from it.

There is little doubt that risk from iron fortification is associated with 'iron overload', and obviously, the higher the intake of dietary iron and the better its availability to the body, the more iron is retained and stored. In normal individuals this leads to an increase in the size of the iron stores and as these increase, absorption of iron is reduced, so a balance is achieved. Nevertheless, in some people an increased amount of iron can cause a disease characterized by extensive and undesirable iron deposits in the liver, heart, pancreas, spleen, and skin. This iron storage disease (known as haemochromatosis) is fortunately rare, affecting only one person in 10,000. However its link with iron fortification is still controversial, and the Swedish study referred to above could not prove any connection.

—Recommended Daily Amounts (RDA) of iron—

The first comprehensive publication of the report on

recommended daily intakes of nutrients for the UK appeared in 1969. These were defined as 'the amounts sufficient or more than sufficient for the nutritional needs of practically all healthy persons in a population'. In the case of iron, for example, this was interpreted as meaning that, in order to maintain health, each person should receive the recommended amount or more. In other words the amount recommended was taken to be a minimum. However, experience has shown that the distribution of nutrient intakes in a group of healthy people is not such that many individuals eat less than the amounts put forward in the 1969 recommendations (DHSS Report on Health and Social Subjects, 15, [HMSO] entitled Recommended Daily Amounts of Food Energy and Nutrients for Groups of People in the United Kingdom) without any recognizable signs of deficiency. A more practical definition of the recommended amount of a nutrient is as follows: the average amount of the nutrient which should be provided per head in a group of people if the needs of practically all members of the group are to be met.

RDAs relate to groups of healthy people. They do not cover any additional needs arising from disease such as infections, disorders or the gastro-intestinal tract (which can reduce the absorption of iron), or abnormalities in the metabolism. Nor is any account taken of the wastage of iron that can occur in wholesale or retail distribution or in kitchen preparation and cooking.

How is the figure arrived at? The RDA of iron is derived from estimates of nutrient requirements, and that of an individual for iron is the amount needed daily to maintain health. Below this level signs of deficiency may develop, and in the case of iron they usually take the form of anaemia. Requirements differ from one individual to another, and an individual's requirements may change with alterations in the composition and nature of the diet as a whole. This is because such alterations may affect the efficiency with which iron is absorbed and utilized.

The requirement of iron is usually worked out to a dietary intake expressed as mg per megajoule (MJ). A megajoule is 1,000 Kilojoules or 243 Kilocalories. Food in the UK provides between 1.1mg and 1.3mg per MJ, and to suggest a figure higher than this would not be practical. It is estimated that on average about 10 per cent of iron in the British diet is absorbed, so it is unlikely that more than 1.3mg is actually assimilated.

For men the recommended amount is 10mg per day, and a diet that contained 1.3mg iron/MJ would supply at least this amount for adult men at all ages and degrees of activity. In men who are active and have high energy intakes there is no need for the additional foods which supply the extra iron to be rich in the mineral.

Women who are past child-bearing age (i.e. they have ceased menstruating) in theory need only 8mg per day. However, the recommendation is set at 10mg per day in order to make up for possible previous iron depletion. Any diet containing 1.3mg iron/MJ would provide this amount as long as the diet satisfied the recommended amounts of energy for women of this age (1,900 Kcals).

The UK RDA for menstruating women is 12mg iron per day. In theory this should be supplied by a diet that satisfied the recommendation for energy (2,150 Kcals) and would meet the needs of all women of this age group except about 10 per cent who have large menstrual losses. The figures for energy and iron intake in both groups of women should, however, be suspected when unsupervised slimming regimes are undertaken since the conventional 1,000 Kcal per day diet is unlikely to provide the necessary iron unless extreme care is taken over food item selection.

During pregnancy, the recommended daily amount of food energy is increased from 9 to 10 MJ during the second and third trimesters (thirds). Assuming the proportion of iron in the diet is unchanged, the amount of dietary iron will increase from 11.7mg to 13.0mg per day. This should be sufficient, but some women do become anaemic and need supplementation with iron.

In nursing mothers, the amount of iron lost in the milk is rather less than the usual menstrual loss and in most cases can be made good by a diet containing 1.3mg iron/MJ. However, during lactation the recommended amount of energy eaten is increased to 11.5 MJ so that if this food contains 1.3mg iron/MJ, it will provide 15mg of the mineral, which is taken as the RDA.

New-born babies will have stores of iron (assuming the iron status of the mother during pregnancy was satisfactory) which

Table 7 Recommended dietary intakes or daily amounts of iron around the world (in milligrams)

Country (year)	Infants		Children			Adult males					Adult females					Pregnant	Lactating
Age (years)	0–0.5	0.5–1.0	1–3	4–6	7–10	11–14	15–18	19–22	23–50	51+	11–14	15–18	19–22	23–50	51+		
West Pacific countries (1980)	5	5	5	5	5	9	5	5	5	5	12	14	14	14	14	14	14
Venezuela (1976)	10	10	10	10	10	18	9	9	9	9	24	28	28	28	9	—	—
USSR (1980)	7	7	8	8	8	15	15	18	18	18	15	15	18	18	18	18	18
USA (1980)	10	15	15	10	10	18	18	18	10	10	18	18	18	18	10	—	—
Uruguay (1977)	—	15	10	10	10	18	10	10	10	10	18	18	18	18	10	18	18
UK (1979)	6	6	7	8	10	12	12	10	10	10	12	12	12	13	10	13	15
Turkey (1975)	5	8	8	9	10	12	15	7	7	7	20	23	23	23	10	25	20
Thailand (1970)	1/kg	1/kg	4	4	4	11	11	6	6	6	16	16	16	16	6	26	26
Taiwan (1980)	6	7	8	8	10	15	15	10	10	10	18	18	15	15	15	—	—
Sweden (1980)			—			10	18	18	18	18	18	18	18	18	18	—	—
Spain (1980)	3	5	10	10	10	15	15	15	15	15	15	15	15	15	15	20	25
Singapore (post 1975)	7	7	7	7	7	12	6	6	6	6	18	19	19	19	6	19	19
Romania (1980)	—	—				12	12	12	12	12	20	20	20	20	20	—	—
Portugal (1978)	5	7	8	10	15	15	13	13	13	15	15	15	13	13	—	—	
Poland (1969)			6	7	10	15	15	12	12	12	15	15	12	12	12	15	18
Philippines (1977)	—	9	8	8	7	11	13	10	10	10	18	18	18	19	8	18	18
Norway (1980)						10	10	10	10	10	27	18	18	18	18	—	—
New Zealand (1983)	6	6	7	10	10	12	12	10	10	10	12	12	12	12	12	15	13
Netherlands (1978)	—	1/kg	7	8	10	12	15	10	10	10	12	15	10	10	10	15	15
Mexico (1970)	10	15	15	10	10	18	18	10	10	10	18	18	18	18	10	25	25
Malaysia (1973)	10	10	10	10	10	18	18	9	9	9	24	28	28	28	9	—	—
Korea (1980)	10	15	15	10	10	10	10	10	10	10	18	18	18	18	10	—	—
Japan (1979)	6	6	8	8	9	10	12	10	10	10	12	12	12	12	12	17	20
Italy (1978)	7	7	7	9	9	12	15	10	10	10	18	18	18	18	10	18	18
Indonesia (1980)	10	10	10	10	10	15	15	9	9	9	12	24	28	12	12	30	32
India (1981)	1/kg	1/kg	22.5	22.5	22.5	25	24	24	24	22.5	35	32	32	32	40	32	
Cen. America & Panama (1973)	5	10	10	10	10	10	18	9	9	9	10	24	24	28	28	28	28
Hungary (1978)	7	7	7	7	7	12	12	12	9	9	18	18	18	9	9	19	19
East Germany (1980)	6	6	8	8	10	10	12	12	10	10	15	15	15	15	10	20	20
West Germany (1975)	6	8	8	8	10	12	12	12	12	12	18	18	18	18	10	25	20
France (1981)	—	—	10	10	10	10	10	15	10	10	10	18	18	18	18	20	20
Finland (1980)	5	5	5	5	5	9	5	5	5	5	12	14	14	14	5	14	14
FAO/WHO (1974)	7.5	7.5	7.5	7.5	7.5	7.5	7	7	7	7	7.5	21	21	21	21	—	—
Denmark (1985)	10	10	10	18	18	18	18	18	18	18	27	27	27	27	27	—	—
Czechoslovakia (1981)	5	8	8	9	12	13	15	12	12	12	15	17	14	14	14	18	21
Colombia (1975)	4	8	8	8	11	14	9	9	9	16	22	22	22	9	27	24	
China (1981)	10	10	10	10	10	15	15	12	12	21	18	18	15	15	15	36	18
Chile (1978)	10	10	10	10	10	18	18	10	12	12	18	18	18	18	15	36	—
Caribbean (1976)	5	5	7	7	7	12	6	6	6	6	16	19	19	19	6	19	19
Canada (1975)	7	7	8	9	10	9	12	10	10	10	10	11	9	9	9	14	18
Bulgaria (1980)	6.5	8.5	12	13	14	15	14	16	13	13	15	18	22	19	19	23	24
Bolivia (1968)	4	5	8	8	8	14	14	7	7	7	18	18	21	21	6	27	23
Australia (1970)	—	4.8	5	7	10	12	12	10	7	7	12	12	12	12	12	15	15
Argentina (1976)	7.5	7.5	7.5	7.5	7.5	7.5	7	7	7	7	18	21	21	21	21	—	—

together with the iron present in human milk can satisfy requirements for the first four to six months. Thereafter supplementary feeding usually begins and the increased needs should be adequately met. Experience indicates that if children consume diets providing 1.3mg iron/MJ their requirements are likely to be met and they are unlikely to become anaemic. The RDAs for both adolescent boys and girls are 12mg to allow for growth in the males and menstrual loss in the females.

These, then, are the reasonings behind the assessment of RDAs of iron by the authorities in the UK. However, as Table 7 indicates, different figures for different countries suggest that there are uncertainties for those nutrients that require judgement. In the case of iron, committees differ concerning the feasibility of covering women with the highest 5 per cent of menstrual losses by advising very high iron intakes for everyone.

Some of the figures in Table 7 are average values since in some countries different intakes are recommended depending upon physical activity. Where figures for pregnant and lactating females are not given, it is usually because the authorities have concluded that the increased requirements are not attainable from the diet and supplementation with iron is essential. For example, in the USA, the use of 30 to 60mg of supplemental iron is recommended during pregnancy. Although it is believed by the authorities that iron needs during lactation are not substantially different from those of non-pregnant women, they recommend continued supplementation of the mother for two to three months after giving birth in order to replenish stores of the mineral depleted by pregnancy. The high figures recommended by India reflect the largely vegetarian nature of the diet of most of the population and take account of the reduced availability of iron from vegetable sources.

CHAPTER 3

The Functions of Iron in the Body

Iron is present in all cells of the body and therefore plays a key role in several biochemical reactions. One of the most important is that of a carrier of oxygen as a constituent of haemoglobin (the red pigment of blood), myoglobin (the red pigment of muscle), and several coenzymes called cytochromes that function in the body to, amongst other things, maintain physical work performance.

The way in which the body maintains iron balance and prevents the development of iron deficiency is the result of three unique mechanisms. These are as follows:

1. A continuous reutilization of iron from cells that are broken down when their useful life is finished.
2. The presence of a specific storage protein called ferritin which allows iron to be stored in the body to meet any future extra demand, for example in pregnancy.
3. The regulation of the absorption of iron. This is affected by actual requirements — there is increased absorption of the mineral when iron is deficient and decreased absorption when iron is present in excessive amounts.

In spite of these ingenious mechanisms for the conservation of iron and in view of the fact that, as we have seen, iron is present in a wide variety of foods, the apparently moderate requirements of the mineral are not always met. The fact remains that iron deficiency is the most prevalent mineral deficiency in the world. We shall now look at the factors that may contribute to this state of affairs and discuss body iron and its turnover.

Iron metabolism

An adult male contains about 4 grams of iron in his body and an adult female contains about 2.5 grams. The major part of the iron is present as haem complexes in haemoglobin, myoglobin, and a number of haem-containing enzymes. Haemoglobin is the red oxygen-carrying pigment present in the red blood cells; myoglobin is the oxygen-carrying pigment in muscle that gives meat its red colour, and the haem-containing enzymes function as oxygen carriers within the body cells. In addition to these haem-containing enzymes, iron is also present in the tissues as non-haem enzymes such as certain oxidases and other enzymes where iron is a cofactor.

Iron is stored as two protein complexes called ferritin and haemosiderin. The richest storage depots are in the organs, especially the liver, spleen, and bone-marrow. These are all rich-red in colour, and this reflects the high concentration of the stored iron in them. In adult men the body stores can amount to 1,000mg, but in women the stores are much nearer 300mg and seldom exceed 500mg. Many studies have indicated that a large proportion of women in both industrialized and developing countries have no iron stores at all.

Table 8 Approximate amounts of iron-containing compounds in the body

Form	Iron compounds	75kg male (mg)	55kg female (mg)
Functional compounds	Haemoglobin	2,300	1,700
	Myoglobin	320	220
	Haem enzymes	80	50
	Non-haem enzymes	100	60
	Iron in transport	3	3
		2,803	2,033
Storage complexes	Ferritin	700	200
	Haemosiderin	300	70
		1,000	270
	TOTAL	3,803	2,303

The way in which iron is distributed in the male and female body is illustrated in Table 8. The figures are taken from the classic publication by T. H. Bothwell, R. W. Charlton, J. D. Cook, and C. A. Finch, *Iron Metabolism in Man* (Blackwell, 1979).

When iron is transported from the storage depots to tissues where it is needed, it is carried 'complexed' to a specific protein in the blood plasma called transferrin. In its storage and transport complexes with protein iron is always present in the ferric form. Binding with protein is essential since iron in the free ionic or salt form is highly toxic within the blood and tissues of the body. It is because iron is bound with protein and is not in the ionic or salt form that it is not excreted by the kidney and hence does not appear in the urine.

————How iron is cycled within the body————

There are two distinct cycles or loops of iron metabolism which we can regard for convenience as an internal and an external or outer loop. The internal loop consists of a continuous reutilization of iron derived from red blood cells that have reached the end of their life. It is this zealous retention of used iron and its incorporation into new red blood cells that are of very great importance in maintaining haemoglobin levels in the blood. The external loop represents losses of iron from the body, which we shall deal with in detail later, and its absorption from the diet.

Let us now look at the important internal loop. Red blood cells live for about 120 days and then, by some unknown mechanism, the cells of that age are plucked from the bloodstream as they pass through the spleen. The spleen contains specialized cells that make up the reticuloendothelial system, and it is these cells that possess the ability to destroy old red blood cells. During the destructive process, haemoglobin is released and this in turn is degraded to its constituent parts, iron, protein, and haem. The protein is digested and broken down into its simple amino acids; haem becomes bile pigments and iron is bound by the blood plasma protein transferrin.

Hence, still attached to tranferrin, iron is transported to the bone-marrow, which is the site at which the mineral is incorporated into haemoglobin and thence into new red blood cells. Some of this iron, of course, is used in the formation of these cells and some finds its way to the various storage components throughout the body. Nevertheless the main part of the internal iron metabolism is a recycling operation to produce the mineral for new blood cell mass. The external loop will be discussed in greater detail later when we talk about iron requirements and its absorption.

These iron exchanges have been measured by Dr C. V. Moore, who used the technique of radioactive tracers of iron to follow the movement of the mineral within the body. His results were presented in a series of lectures in the Harvey lecture series of 1959-60.

If we assume a daily dietary intake of 12mg iron, 1mg is absorbed and the remaining 11mg is lost in the faeces. In one day, the turnover of iron in the blood plasma is about 35mg, 1mg of which is that absorbed from the food, the remainder being supplied from the breakdown of old red blood cells (20mg) and from iron stores (14mg). A total of 1mg is lost daily in cells sloughed from the skin, gastro-intestinal tract, and urinary systems, and in theory this is replaced by the 1mg absorbed from the diet. To this loss must be added an extra 28mg iron present in the menstrual flow in females. As we shall see, this is ideally but not always replaced by extra absorption from the food.

──────────Iron losses from the body──────────

In an ideal situation, iron absorbed from the food will exactly replace that lost from the body via various routes. At the same time, body storage levels will be maintained so that reserves can be called upon when losses are heavy, for instance in the menstrual flow, in haemorrhage, and after childbirth. It is impossible to replace such losses immediately from the diet, so iron reserves will maintain functional levels until a slow build-up can eventually replenish these. The menstrual flow may last 5 days, but it is during the 28 days or so of the cycle that extra iron must be eaten to make up for the losses.

Let us now consider how iron is lost to the body during normal physiological processes. To these must be added extra losses that will occur during certain illnesses. Whilst acute losses that are serious are normally replaced quickly by blood transfusion, long-term insidious losses may not be so obvious, but nevertheless iron intake must increase to allow for them.

Basal iron losses

Iron is present in all body cells, so when these are lost by normal sloughing off, the iron in them is irretrievably lost also. The cells we lose constantly are mainly from the skin and gastro-intestinal tract and the iron in them has been calculated to be 14µg/kg body weight daily, which works out at about 1.0mg in a 70kg man and 0.8mg in a 55kg woman. These low-weight, but, in terms of iron, significant losses were measured accurately by giving radioactive iron intravenously to human volunteers. After about one year to allow the radioactive mineral to be mixed with the blood, tissues, and storage forms, the amount of iron secreted daily was calculated from the decrease in radioactivity of haemoglobin iron over two years. These precise measurements were reported in 1968 by Drs R. Green, R. W. Charlton, and H. Seftel in the *American Journal of Medicine* and they confirmed the degree of regular losses that had been suspected for many years.

At one time daily iron losses by excessive sweating were considered to be significant and athletes were suspected of losing several milligrams of iron via this route during their strenuous training and competition. Now this is no longer accepted since a study in Dar es Salaam on the effect of work level and dietary intake on the secretion of iron and other minerals in a hot climate. The active young men in the study were found to lose only between 250 and 500µg of iron daily. Although this represents a loss of up to half a milligram, it is far less than had been expected, and of course the exercise undertaken by the subjects in the trial was far beyond the norm. Sweating will cause some iron loss, but in most people this is insignificant compared to that lost normally via the body cell loss.

On these measurements, men should therefore absorb at least 1mg of iron daily from the diet and women 0.8mg simply to replace a loss over which they have no control. However, women of child-bearing age have additional losses because of menstruation, so these must be taken into consideration when calculating ideal dietary intakes of the mineral.

─────────Menstrual iron losses─────────

Basal iron losses are suffered by all sectors of the population, but in the female must be added iron lost in the menstrual flow and that lost to the foetus during pregnancy. What has emerged from many studies is the fact that menstrual iron losses are constant in every cycle in a particular woman, but can vary tremendously between different women. It is for this reason that some women have much greater iron requirements than others.

Two large studies have been undertaken to determine how much iron a woman loses in her menstrual flow. One was carried out in Britain by Drs A. Jacobs and E. B. Butler and reported in *The Lancet* in 1965; the other came from Sweden, was the result of trials carried out by Drs L. Hallberg, A. M. Hogdall, L. Nilsson, and G. Rybo, and was reported in the *Swedish Medical Journal* in 1966. All the women were randomly selected from the general population.

It was found that most women lost between 20 and 40ml of blood each period. Since their blood on average contained 12.5 grams haemoglobin per 100ml, the actual haemoglobin lost was between 2.5 and 5 grams. Haemoglobin contains about 0.34 per cent iron, so that each lost gram is associated with a depletion of 3.4mg of the mineral. Hence the iron lost in menstruation can range from 8.5 to 17.0mg. To replace these losses over the whole 28-day menstrual cycle, an extra 0.3 to 0.6mg of iron per day must be absorbed. Although losses occur over a 5-day period, replenishment takes longer and ideally should be complete by the start of the next menstrual flow.

These figures, however, apply only to the lower end of menstrual losses. In 25 per cent of the women studied their menstrual flow was heavier and longer and their iron losses averaged over the whole of the cycle were 0.9mg per day compared to the more normal 0.6mg per day. Ten per cent of the women in the study lost more than 80ml of blood at each period, culminating in a loss of iron exceeding 1.4mg per day. If we add to this the basal iron losses of 0.8mg daily, it can be seen that these 10 per cent of menstruating women have total iron requirements, necessary to replace all losses, of 2.2mg per day taken over the whole of the menstrual cycle. It is not hard to imagine the difficulties for these women in achieving such intakes when, as we shall see, iron is notoriously difficult to absorb. Perhaps it is not surprising that in many women, mild anaemia is the norm rather than the exception.

The figures we have discussed refer to a 55kg (121 lb, 8.5 stone) woman. Logically, menstrual iron losses are related to the size of the uterus whence the menstrual flow comes, and it can be expected that the greater the weight of the female, the larger the uterus. Hence in populations where the females are bigger and heavier than 55kg menstrual iron losses can be considerably higher than those quoted, and conversely, in populations where the women are of smaller stature, losses would be expected to be less. This fact should be considered in assessing iron requirements in different populations.

In addition, other factors that may influence iron lost in the menstrual flow should be considered. Those women who take the contraceptive pill tend to produce thinner linings of the uterus (the endometrium), so their menstrual losses of iron are about half those of comparable women who do not practise this form of contraception. If a woman use the intrauterine contraceptive device (the coil), her menstrual losses are likely to increase to about 50 per cent over those in comparable women not using them. This is because the local irritant effect of the coil does appear to cause extra bleeding over and above that due to breakdown of the normal-size endometrium.

Pregnancy and lactation

The loss of iron involved during a normal pregnancy and the ensuing period of lactation is contributed to by a number of factors. First there is the basal loss of 0.8mg daily which adds up, during the 270 days of pregnancy, to about 220mg. The growing foetus takes up 400mg iron, all provided by the mother and so lost to her. The placenta and uterus have an iron content of 125mg, and during delivery, the normal blood loss will cause a further depletion of 200mg iron. The total iron requirements during pregnancy can thus be estimated as about 1,000mg since this amount is lost to the mother.

During the lactation or breast-feeding period there are the usual basal losses of 0.8mg iron per day, to which must be added the iron lost into breast milk, about 0.25mg per day. This totals just more than 1mg daily, so over the six months of breast-feeding, an extra 180mg of iron is needed to replace that provided in the milk.

On the positive side, menstrual losses cease during the periods of pregnancy and lactation, and as these total about 450 days (approximately 15 months), 255mg of iron is saved. There is still a shortfall of about 750mg iron, and this can only be replaced by an extra absorption of about 1.7mg daily averaged over the total period of 450 days. Not surprisingly, diet is often unable to supply the extra mineral to make up the deficit.

It has been calculated that in most pregnancies there is a shortfall between intake and losses of about 200mg iron. If stores of the mineral are at this figure then they can be temporarily drawn upon. Too often, however, the mother has virtually no stores, so she is bound to develop iron-deficient anaemia that will only respond to supplementation with the mineral. These figures were calculated for a female of 55kg non-pregnant weight so if she weighs more than this, iron needs must also increase. This variation in body weight of different populations probably accounts for the wide range of RDAs suggested during pregnancy that are shown in Table 7.

A great problem is that the enhanced requirements of iron during pregnancy are not evenly distributed over the whole period. They develop mainly in the second half or third trimester of pregnancy because this is when the rate of growth of the foetus is greatest. It is not unusual for the total iron requirements of the mother to be 7-8mg per day during the last month of pregnancy. There is no way that these requirements can be met by diet alone. Hence it is reasonable to imagine that a main function of iron stores in the body is to counteract the development of iron deficiency in the latter part of pregnancy.

Clinical studies indicate that there is no increase in the absorption of iron from the diet during the early part of pregnancy when the iron requirements are low. As they increase during the later stages of pregnancy so does the efficiency of absorption, so there is some compensation for the extra needs during this period.

It has been calculated that iron stores of 500mg are needed to balance the iron requirements during pregnancy, but such an ideal is rarely found in modern young women: hence the almost standard practice of taking iron supplements during the second half of pregnancy. Such an approach reflects the present low dietary intake of energy and iron in women of industrialized countries. To this must be added the low bioavailability of iron from the diets of those living in the developing countries. Little wonder, then, that iron deficiency during pregnancy is a world-wide problem.

Iron intake and growth

When born, the full-term infant has iron stores sufficient to cover its requirements for the first four to six months. Once these have gone, the iron requirements for growth must be met entirely by the diet. During the first year of life the average infant triples its body weight and at the same time almost doubles its body content of iron.

An infant of six months needs to absorb from 0.5 to 0.8mg of iron per day to supply its requirements. This amount of iron is very high in relation to the infant's energy intake. However, at the breast-feeding stage human milk remains virtually the sole source of iron for the infant. Breast milk supplies only about 0.25mg iron per day, but this iron is in an extremely well-absorbed form (about 50 per cent), so the actual quantity assimilated by the baby is about 0.1mg per day. Whilst this is a useful contribution to the baby's iron needs, most of these will be provided by its body stores.

Iron in cow's milk is for some unknown reason less well absorbed than that in human milk. It is therefore usual for manufacturers of dried baby milks (whether produced from cow's or goat's milk) to add iron salts to their product to augment the iron to a level which will give a comparable absorbed amount to that in human milk. What dried baby milks lack in quality of iron they make up for in quantity. In addition, once weaning starts, significant amounts of iron are supplied by the cereals that are usually introduced at this time, and since these too may be fortified with the mineral, the requirements of the infant are probably met.

Premature infants and those of low birth weight should have extra iron supplied to them at an early stage in their lives according to a report in the *American Journal of Nutrition* in 1980. This is because the body stores of these babies are lower than normal. In all infants, however, the critical period with the highest risk of iron deficiency is between 6 months and 2 years of age. Thereafter the demand for iron decreases as the rate of body growth slows.

During childhood, then, the daily requirements for absorbed iron decreases to between 0.5 and 0.8mg daily, but at the onset of adolescence, when growth spurts again, the needs increase to between 0.5 and 1.0mg daily. An adolescent girl will need iron to allow for her basal losses and menstrual losses plus that required for her increased haemoglobin and body mass, both of which increase as she approaches adulthood.

We can conclude, therefore, that iron deficiency due to low intakes is a common problem throughout childhood, particularly in developing countries but by no means confined to them. At all levels of society, because of the resistance to particular foods and a propensity to faddy diets that occur during childhood, children are at risk of low iron intakes. As we have seen, these can not only lead to restricted physical growth, but to reduced mental development. The net result is a high risk of developing iron deficiency that is extended over the whole pre-school period and often beyond it.

————Other non-medical losses of iron————

A blood donation of 400 to 450ml represents an iron loss of about 200mg, and this can only be replaced by an increased iron absorption of 0.5mg per day over one year. Anyone who donates more than this amount per year will therefore have a very high iron requirement and they should be aware of the need to obtain this in their diet. As an example, men who donate blood six times a year will have an extra iron requirement of 3mg daily on top of their basal losses of 1mg, giving a total amount of 4mg per day that must be absorbed to prevent deficiency. A woman who gives blood four times a year will have to absorb a total of 3.4mg iron per day to make up her basal and menstrual losses in addition to those lost in the donated blood. Blood donation should present no problems to any healthy adult as long as their diet is such as to replace the lost iron. Anyone with good body stores of iron will in no way compromise their iron status by regular but not-too-frequent donations of blood. Supplementation will of course replace iron stores more rapidly.

Medical losses of iron

These fall into three categories:

Acute haemorrhage

The sudden loss of at least one litre of blood from a wound or from post-delivery or intestinal bleeding induces shock, also known as peripheral circulatory failure. If rapid losses of two or three litres of blood occur, the result is usually fatal, but the body can cope with such losses if spread over a longer period, say one or two days. What happens then is that the blood volume is maintained by the withdrawal of tissue fluid which is then introduced into the blood. The volume is restored but at the expense of thinner blood. For example, blood containing 15g of haemoglobin per 100ml will, after the rapid loss of one litre of it, contain only 12g of haemoglobin per 100ml. By dietary means alone this blood would take a very long time to be restored to its previous haemoglobin content. For this reason, blood transfusion is virtually essential for fast replacement of blood and of course iron lost during acute haemorrhage.

Chronic haemorrhage

This is usually less obvious than acute haemorrhage, and its often insidious nature can gradually induce a mild to serious loss of iron from the body. Losses may be small and constant or regularly repetitive, depending on their cause. Typical are menorrhagia (abnormally heavy bleeding at menstruation) in females and bleeding from the gastro-intestinal tract in both sexes. This may result from cancer, gastric and duodenal ulceration, haemorrhoids (piles), ulcerative colitis, and diverticulitis. One significant cause of persistent blood loss is the regular taking of high-dose aspirin (e.g. by those suffering from arthritis) and other anti-inflammatory drugs. Anyone with these conditions should be aware of a potential steady iron loss from the body because of them and must look to their dietary intake of the mineral, possibly with supplementation.

Hookworm infection

In areas where certain parasitic infections, especially hookworm, are prevalent, additional iron is required to replace the increased intestinal losses of blood. Infection with hookworm is a common cause of anaemia where there is 'wet' cultivation of the land. What happens is that haemorrhages occur at the site of attachment of the worms to the intestinal mucous membrane. Each worm may ingest from 0.03 to 0.15ml of blood daily. Anyone therefore with a high infestation of worms (about 1,000) is going to lose 30 to 150ml of blood daily, equivalent to heavy menstrual losses of iron. Anaemia will therefore develop quickly. Even mild infestation of worms will cause an insidious loss of blood (and hence iron) that will have to be replaced. These studies were carried out in West Africa and Venezuela, where the problem was exacerbated by the low dietary intake of iron in the indigenous population.

───────────The absorption of iron───────────

The absorption of iron from the diet is influenced by a variety of factors that include the amount and form of the dietary iron; the presence of dietary factors enhancing absorption; the presence of dietary factors inhibiting absorption; and the iron status of the body. We shall now consider each factor in turn and try to assess the extent of its influence in determining how much iron is absorbed and the possible contribution to iron deficiency.

───────────Two dietary forms of iron───────────

As explained in Chapter 2 there are two kinds of iron in the diet, haem and non-haem iron, and they differ in their extent of absorption. The mechanism of absorption is the reason why haem iron is taken up by the absorbing cells of the intestine (called mucosal cells) intact, but once it is inside the cell a haem-splitting enzyme separates the iron from the accompanying carrier. Another carrier protein within the cell then transfers the iron to the other side of the cell adjacent to the blood system whence it is carried to other parts of the body.

Non-haem iron cannot be absorbed from the diet intact because it must first be separated from the substance with which it is combined (called a ligand). It is the shedding of ligands that creates problems, but once they are gone, the iron left is in the ionic or positively charged form. Because it is positively charged, ionic iron tends to stick to the walls of the intestine, which are negatively charged. Eventually, however, specific receptors in the intestinal cell manage to pluck the ionic iron into the cell, where it ends up as an iron-protein (or amino-acid) complex. Once inside the intestinal (or mucosal) cell, this complex is treated in exactly the same way as the haem iron-protein complex referred to above. Thereafter, transfer from the mucosal cell into the circulating blood is carried out in the same way for both types of iron.

It is in the absorption from the food into the mucosal cells of the intestine that the essential difference between haem iron and non-haem iron lies. The absorption of non-haem iron is markedly affected by the iron status of the individual, which results in greater absorption of the mineral in those who are iron-deficient. On the other hand, the extent of absorption of haem iron at low levels bears no relationship to the amount of iron the subject already has. Haem iron in a few milligrams' concentration is absorbed regardless.

Another difference between the two types of iron is that the absorption of non-haem iron is significantly affected by a great number of factors in the diet. Some, like phytic acid, present in cereals, tea, and coffee inhibit its absorption, but others, such as vitamin C, meat, and fish, enhance the absorption of non-haem iron. Haem iron is unaffected by all these factors, but there is some evidence that the presence of meat in the diet enhances even the absorption of this type of iron.

When we look at the diets of developing countries we find that the content of haem iron is usually negligible. In the average western-type diet, which contains between 10 and 20mg of iron in total (i.e. about 6–7mg per 1,000Kcal), haem iron contributes only between 1 and 2mg iron per day despite the high meat consumption. The absorption of haem iron in meals containing meat is about 25 per cent in both iron-replete and iron-deficient subjects. When eaten without meat, haem iron added to a meal is absorbed only to the extent of about 10 per cent. In a mixed diet, however, the absorption of non-haem iron is somewhat less than 10 per cent.

At high intakes of haem iron, there is a degree of control of absorption depending upon the amount in the diet and the iron status of the person. Hence if black pudding (blood sausage) is eaten as part of a meal, it provides between 40 and 50mg iron, and at this level absorption of the mineral decreases to about 2.5 per cent. This reduced level of assimilation also occurs if the person is already overloaded with iron. Conversely, if the individual is deficient, the extent of absorption of haem iron will increase accordingly.

As the above figures indicate, non-haem iron is the main source of iron even in a mixed diet; in the vegan and vegetarian diets it is the sole source. Since non-haem iron is the type most affected by other factors in the diet, the variation in iron absorption between different meals and diets is mainly related to a variation in the absorption of that non-haem iron.

One other factor that determines the absorbability of non-haem iron is gastric acid. Normally hydrochloric acid is present in the digestive juices of the stomach, and it is now known that gastric hydrochloric acid facilitates the absorption of non-haem iron by converting ferric to ferrous iron. When this stomach acid is missing—the condition known as achlorhydria—the absorption of iron decreases dramatically. Hence there appears to be a relationship between achlorhydria and iron-defiency anaemia, and it has been demonstrated that lack of gastric acid reduces absorption of food iron by about 50 per cent.

————How absorption of iron is measured————

The major problem in measuring food iron uptake is the wide variability in absorption. A large factor in this is subject-to-subject variation. This makes it difficult to determine to what extent differences in absorption between different meals, studied in different groups of subjects, relate to the meals and to the iron status of the subjects. The problem may be solved by determining in each subject the absorption both from the meal studied and from a measured dose of an iron salt given under the standard fasting conditions. An absorption of 40 per cent from the reference dose is taken as the standard or normalized absorption. If for example, in a test on an individual 20 per cent of the reference dose of iron and 4 per cent of the food iron were absorbed, the normalized absorption from the meal would be taken as 8 per cent (i.e. twice the observed absorption because 40 per cent is twice 20 per cent). A level of 40 per cent absorption value is taken because it is representative of borderline iron-deficiency subjects who have no iron stores but no anaemia either. It is therefore of special significance in calculating iron balances.

How is it possible to distinguish absorbed iron from that already there? As explained in Chapter 2 the answer lies in a method of tagging or marking the iron in the diet so that it can be measured and separated from inherent iron, and the best way to tag iron is to make it radioactive. Radioactivity is readily measured and any radioactive iron within the blood or tissues of the body can only have got there through absorption, so a measure of this is then obtained. The whole technique depends upon the fact that radioactive iron is treated by the body like any other iron, and once absorbed it joins the general pool of the mineral in the body and soon equilibrates with it.

This technique is a research tool, but it can be applied as a diagnostic test to determine, for example, if a person is able to absorb iron efficiently. It has been invaluable in studying the absorption of iron from individual items of food; from whole meals and from supplementary forms of the mineral. It has told us also that individuals vary tremendously in the extent to which they absorb iron. It enables other factors in food to be studied for their effect on iron absorption, for example the extent to which vitamin C and meat enhance absorption and the extent to which phytic acid can inhibit absorption.

One of the first studies utilizing this technique measured the absorption of iron from individual foods as it was carried out on 87 Venezuelan peasants by Drs M. Layrisse and C. Martinez-Torres and reported in *Progress in Haematology* in 1971. Radioactive iron was incorporated into proteins of animal origin by injecting it into the animal and allowing it time to become part of the animal's tissues before slaughter. In this way the absorption of haem iron was measured. The results of these pioneering studies are shown in Table 9 and the information supplied by them is invaluable.

The percentage absorption is an average figure, but there was a wide variation in the cases studied. Without exception, these studies indicated that iron in foods of animal origin is better absorbed than that in vegetables. This is why in communities where 70 per cent or more of the energy intake comes from whole

Table 9 Iron absorption from different foods

Vegetable foods	No. of cases studied	Dose of iron (mg)	% absorbed
Rice	11	2	1.0
Spinach	9	2	1.4
Black beans	137	3–4	3.0
Maize	73	2–4	3.5
Lettuce	13	1–17	4.0
Wheat	42	2–4	5.0
Soya beans	38	3–4	7.0
Animal origin foods			
Ferritin	17	3	7.6
Veal liver	11	3	15.0
Fish muscle	34	1–2	12.0
Haemoglobin	39	3–4	13.0
Veal muscle	96	3–4	20.0

wheat, maize, and sorghum, daily intakes of iron may be up to 20mg and yet iron deficiency is widespread. The poor absorption of the mineral from these vegetables is probably exacerbated by the presence of phytic acid in them.

The information in the tables illustrates the marked variety in the absorption of iron from different meals and indicates the actual amount that is bioavailable. Only a minor part of the variation can be ascribed to different non-haem iron contents of the meals. There is a small amount of haem iron in some of the meals, and absorption of this has been assessed at 25 per cent.

The iron absorption from the breakfasts varied from 0.07 to 0.40mg iron. The absorption from the lunches/dinner quoted show a ten-fold variation. It can be seen that iron can be well absorbed from a vegetarian meal when it has a high content of ascorbic acid. In the 1,000Kcal meals there was an almost six-fold difference in the bioavailability of the iron in the presence of food containing the vitamin.

The amount of iron assimilated from diets in developing countries also depends mainly on their content of fish, meat, vitamin C, and fibre. In addition, the choice of drink taken with a meal can markedly influence iron absorption. The extremes are tea and orange juice. Tea is not the only beverage that depresses

Table 10 Iron absorption from breakfast meals

	Iron content		Absorption		Total absorption (mg)
	Non-haem (mg)	Haem (mg)	Non-haem (mg)	Haem (mg)	
Continental breakfast with coffee	2.8	0	0.16	0	0.16
Continental breakfast with coffee plus orange juice	3.1	0	0.40	0	0.40
Continental breakfast with coffee plus boiled egg	4.1	0	0.19	0	0.19
Continental breakfast with coffee plus scrambled egg and bacon	4.2	0.03	0.25	0.01	0.26
Continental breakfast with coffee plus cornflakes and milk	3.6	0	0.16	0	0.16
Continental breakfast with tea	2.8	0	0.07	0	0.07
Continental breakfast with tea plus orange juice	3.1	0	0.21	0	0.21
Continental breakfast with tea plus scrambled egg and bacon	4.2	0.03	0.12	0.01	0.13
Continental breakfast with drinking chocolate	3.2	0	0.11	0	0.11

Table 11 Iron absorption from western-type lunch/dinner dishes

	Iron content		Absorption		Total absorption
	Non-haem (mg)	Haem (mg)	Non-haem (mg)	Haem (mg)	(mg)
Meat meals					
Meat balls, potatoes, jam, milk	2.6	0.5	0.29	0.12	0.41
Spaghetti with meat sauce	2.7	0.6	0.31	0.15	0.46
Pea soup and pork, milk	3.5	0	0.35	0	0.35
Sole au gratin, potatoes	2.1	0	0.38	0	0.38
Hamburger, potatoes, string beans	3.0	0.5	0.38	0.12	0.50
Beans and pork, milk	5.4	0.3	0.43	0.07	0.50
Roast beef, green beans, potatoes	3.1	1.0	0.58	0.25	0.83
Borsch (beetroot soup and meat)	2.8	1.1	0.81	0.27	1.08
Sauerkraut and sausage	2.0	0.6	0.90	0.15	1.05
Cheese, sausage, caviar, and milk	4.0	0	0.32	0	0.32
Vegetarian meals					
Navy beans, brown rice, bread, apple, walnuts, almonds, yogurt, and margarine	5.8	0	0.13	0	0.13
Pancakes, strawberry jam, milk	5.1	0	0.18	0	0.18
Cauliflower, red kidney beans, tomato sauce, bread, margarine, cottage cheese, pineapple, banana	5.8	0	0.98	0	0.98

Table 12 Iron absorption from typical meals with an energy content of about 1,000Kcal

	Iron content		Absorption		Total absorption
	Non-haem (mg)	Haem (mg)	Non-haem (mg)	Haem (mg)	(mg)
Pizza and beer	4.2	0	0.33	0	0.33
Hamburger, bread, ketchup, mustard, chips, milk shake	3.9	1.15	0.48	0.29	0.77
Vegetable soup, rye bread, butter, cheese	7.0	0	0.55	0	0.55
Spaghetti, cheese, ketchup	4.9	0	0.59	0	0.59
Boiled cod, potatoes, bread, butter, cake, beer	7.8	0	0.80	0	0.80
Shrimps, beef, vegetable salad, potato, ice-cream	6.2	1.44	0.94	0.36	1.30
Chicken soup, steak and kidney pie, peas, carrots, bread, butter, beer, jelly	5.7	0.94	1.08	0.23	1.31
Meat, beans, onion, tomatoes, bread, wine	7.2	0.80	1.16	0.20	1.36
Gazpacho, chicken, vegetable flan, bread, wine	7.6	0.10	1.35	0.03	1.38
Antipasta, spaghetti, meat, bread, wine, orange	7.8	0.60	1.80	0.15	1.95

the absorption of non-haem iron; coffee does so to a lesser extent. Alcohol promotes absorption of non-haem iron slightly. Wine can markedly increase the absorption of non-haem iron from a meal, not because of its alcohol content but because most wines, both red and white, have a high iron content.

The main factors that determine the bioavailability of non-haem iron are vitamin C content and the presence of meat and fish. Other factors are the acidity of a meal (for example sauerkraut is very acid); the beverages drunk with a meal; and the amount and type of dietary fibre. We shall now look at these in more detail, quantifying the absorption of iron when this has been measured using the methods discussed above.

———How vitamin C increases the absorption——— of non-haem iron

We have seen how new methodology introducing radioactivity-labelled iron enables the extent of absorption of the mineral or bioavailability to be measured. Long before this, however, several researchers had showed that orange juice or ascorbic acid in pure form in fairly large doses increased the absorption of dietary iron. Dr C. V. Moore was a pioneer in this research as far back as 1951, and he reported his results in *Transactions of the Association of American Physicians*. His studies were confirmed and extended by other workers over the period from 1955 to 1968.

The first study using labelled iron was carried out by Dr M. H. Sayers and his colleague and reported in the *British Journal of Haematology* in 1973. They found that 50mg of ascorbic acid added to a simple meal of maize increased the absorption of non-haem iron four-fold. At a simultaneous intake of 100mg ascorbic acid the amount of iron absorbed in a similar meal was 5.5 times that in the same meal in the absence of added ascorbic acid. In 1974 similar studies by Dr E. Bjorn-Rasmussen and Dr L. Hallberg indicated a three-fold increase in iron absorbed when only 25mg of the vitamin was added. As vitamin C was increased the amount of absorbed iron also steadily increased — at an added level of 200mg of the vitamin, absorption of the iron went up six-fold.

This amount of ascorbic acid was not found necessary to enhance the iron absorption six-fold by Dr M. Layrisse and colleagues. They reported in the *American Journal of Nutrition* in 1974 that only 70mg of the vitamin was needed for this effect on iron absorption from a maize meal. In the case of rice, Dr M. H. Sayers found that absorption of iron from it was increased three to four-fold with the addition of between 50 and 100mg of vitamin C.

These studies were carried out on meatless meals, but Hallberg looked at how effective vitamin C was when added to composite whole meals. The addition of 50mg ascorbic acid to a pizza meal enhanced iron absorption two to three-fold, and this happened in all the individuals studied. When the same amount of ascorbic acid was added to a hamburger, stringed beans, and mashed potato meal, the relative absorption increase was only 50 per cent, but when allowance is made for the haem iron in the hamburger meal the absorption increase in both meals was the same. This indicates that the vitamin only enhances the absorption of non-haem iron. The addition of 25 and 50mg ascorbic acid to a simple South-East Asian type of meal composed of rice, cooked vegetables, and a curry increased the absorption of iron by 50 and 90 per cent respectively.

The effect of adding different amounts of pure vitamin C on the absorption of non-haem iron from various meals is shown in Table 13.

In every case, ascorbic acid increases the bioavailability of the non-haem iron. It can be concluded that an amount of only 25mg of ascorbic acid can increase the absorption of non-aem iron 1.5-to 3-fold. When 50mg of the vitamin is added, the absorption of iron increases about two to three times. A more marked effect (three to five times) is found with the addition of 100mg vitamin C. The vitamin has also been shown to increase iron absorption from infant milk formulae and infant cereals. Even a level of vitamin C of only 20mg can significantly increase iron absorption.

The extent of increase in non-haem iron absorption, like the absorption of iron itself, can vary tremendously amongst individuals. Tables 14 and 15 illustrate this, the first showing uptake of iron from a pizza meal (iron content 4.2mg) with and without 50mg ascorbic acid and the second indicating uptake from a hamburger meal (non-haem iron content 3.0mg) with and without 50mg ascorbic acid.

Table 13 How ascorbic acid affects iron absorption from various meals

Meal type	No. of subjects	Non-haem iron content (mg)	Ascorbic acid added (mg)	Absorption		
				Without (%)	With (%)	With/without
Maize	6	5	25	5.8	13.1	2.3
Maize	6	5	50	6.8	19.5	2.9
Maize	6	5	100	4.8	20.8	4.3
Maize	13	–	70	2.8	15.9	5.7
Rice	12	2.9	50	4.5	13.6	3.0
Rice	7	2.9	100	2.4	7.7	3.2
Rice	8	5.4	60	3.1	11.4	3.7
Rice	12	7.6	100	3.8	11.0	2.9
Semi-synthetic	12	4.1	25	0.8	1.3	1.6
Semi-synthetic	12	4.1	50	0.8	1.9	2.4
Semi-synthetic	12	4.1	100	0.8	3.2	4.0
Meat meal	13	4.1	100	4.1	6.8	1.7
Pizza	10	4.2	50	6.4	13.3	2.3
Hamburger	10	3.0	50	10.8	18.2	1.7
Thai rice	20	1.9	25	8.4	12.7	1.5
Thai rice	16	1.9	50	8.4	16.1	1.9

Table 14 Iron uptake from pizza meal

Subject	Absorption % Without ascorbic acid	With ascorbic acid
1	26	38
2	10	23
3	6	20
4	6	13
5	4	12
6	4	6
7	4	7
8	4	6
9	3	7
10	1	5

Table 15 Iron uptake from a hamburger meal

Subject	Absorption % Without ascorbic acid	With ascorbic acid
1	16	30
2	16	30
3	15	30
4	15	21
5	15	16
6	14	27
7	12	18
8	9	8
9	5	4
10	5	4

All the studies described indicated a positive effect on non-haem iron absorption by pure ascorbic acid added to the meal. However, in terms of normal living and conventional meals it is perhaps more meaningful to determine how eating ascorbic acid-rich foods in the diet can affect iron uptake. It is important to know whether naturally occurring vitamin C compares favourably with the pure material.

Indications that vitamin C-rich foods do increase iron absorption came first in 1974, when Dr Layrisse and his colleagues reported that 150g of pawpaw containing 66mg ascorbic acid when added to a simple maize meal increased iron absorption about six times, i.e. the same as when 70mg pure ascorbic acid was added.

Confirmation comes from Dr Hallberg, who found that the same amount of pawpaw increased iron uptake three to four-fold when added to a Thai rice meal. Without the pawpaw, the iron absorption from the rice meal was higher than that from the maize meal.

A more usual source of vitamin C in the western diet is orange juice, and this too has a marked effect on the absorption of non-haem iron. A glass of orange juice containing 70mg of the vitamin increased the absorption of non-haem iron about 2.5 times from a continental type of breakfast with coffee and about 3 times from a similar type of breakfast served with tea. A similar amount of orange juice increased the non-haem iron absorption just over two-fold in a standard hamburger meal.

Vegetables in a meal also contribute enough vitamin C to enhance the absorption of non-haem iron. A simple vegetable salad of lettuce, green pepper, and tomatoes providing 45mg of the vitamin will increase non-haem iron absorption from the standard hamburger meal at least 1.8 times. Cauliflower containing 70mg ascorbic acid added to the same hamburger meal doubled the uptake of iron. Even when added to vegetarian meals, cauliflower increases iron absorption three-fold. A typical vegetarian meal was beans, maize, and rice.

Table 16 illustrates the effect of adding foods rich in ascorbic acid on the absorption of non-haem iron from various meals. The basal non-haem iron content is that in the meal type; the extra food which contains both iron and vitamin C is described under the food item.

All these studies show that the effects of pure ascorbic acid and of foods containing about the same amount of the vitamin appear to be the same. A two- to three-fold increase in absorption of non-haem iron from a meal can be expected when 50 to 100mg of ascorbic acid is present in or is added to the meal. It is imperative that the vitamin is ingested at the same time as the meal.

————How meat improves the absorption———— of non-haem iron

We have seen that the prime factor in increasing the absorption of non-haem iron is ascorbic acid. A second important factor is the presence of meat or fish in the diet. Despite the fact that both

Table 16 How ascorbic acid-rich foods enhance the non-haem iron of various foods

Meal type	No of subjects	Ascorbic acid-rich food added		Ascorbic acid (mg)	Non-haem iron content (mg)		Absorption of iron with basal meal		Absorption of iron with extra food		Ratio Extra/Basal absorption
		Food item	Amount (g)		Basal	Extra food	%	mg	%	mg	
Breakfast/coffee	12	Orange juice	150	70	2.8	3.1	5.7	0.16	12.9	0.40	2.5
Breakfast/tea	12	Orange juice	150	70	2.8	3.1	2.5	0.07	6.8	0.21	3.0
Maize meal	13	Papaw	150	66	—	—	1.4	—	8.8	—	—
Maize meal with fish	14	Papaw	150	66	—	—	4.6	—	24.7	—	—
Thai rice meal	14	Papaw	150	75	1.9	2.3	7.7	0.14	27.2	0.61	4.4
Beans, rice, maize	10	Cauliflower	125	70	4.4	5.4	3.4	0.15	9.8	0.53	3.5
Vegetarian I	10	Cauliflower	125	70	5.8	6.8	2.2	0.13	4.7	0.32	2.5
Vegetarian II	10	Cauliflower	125	70	5.8	6.8	5.5	0.32	14.7	0.98	3.1
Hamburger	12	Orange juice	150	70	3.0	3.3	8.3	0.29	19.1	0.63	2.2
Hamburger	10	Vegetable salad	145	45	3.0	3.6	8.7	0.26	13.3	0.48	1.8
Hamburger	10	Cauliflower	125	70	3.0	4.0	14.6	0.44	26.4	1.05	2.4

improve the absorption of non-haem iron, the mechanisms involved are different and quite independent. Whereas ascorbic acid has no effect upon the absorption of haem iron, meat seems to increase the uptake of both haem and non-haem iron. Even in their effect upon non-haem iron, both ascorbic acid and meat appear to exert their effort independently, so when eaten together in the same meal their absorption-promoting effects will be additive.

Studies to prove this came from Dr L. Hallberg and L. Rossander and were published in the *American Journal of Clinical Nutrition* in 1981. The studies were carried out on two meals to which meat or fish was added and to and from which cauliflower (rich in ascorbic acid) was added or subtracted. The results are shown in Table 17.

It is of interest that the effect of 90g of meat was less marked than that of 70mg ascorbic acid as cauliflower. The third experiment indicates that meat improves the absorption of added iron also. However, it should be remembered that the effect of meat, fish, and ascorbic acid must to some extent be related to the initial absorption from the meal before adding these enhancing factors. The higher the initial absorption the smaller is the relative effect that can be expected.

————Factors that inhibit iron absorption————

High dietary fibre intake and the beverages coffee and tea are all factors that have been found to reduce non-haem bioavailability from the diet. We shall now consider each in turn to determine the significance of their effect and see how their inhibiting action may be overcome.

——————High dietary fibre intake——————

In 1978 Dr J. L. Kelsay published a review of research on effects of fibre intake in man in the *American Journal of Clinical Nutrition* and concluded that 'a number of reports indicate that mineral absorption is decreased by fibre'. The net effect depends upon a number of parameters amongst which are phytic acid concentration of the fibre, the level of fibre in the diet, and the type of fibre. Fibres are of several different kinds and all differ in their physical and chemical properties and also their mineral-binding capacities.

Table 17 The additive effect of meat and ascorbic acid on iron uptake from vegetarian meals

Meal	Iron uptake from meal (mg)	From meal + meat or fish (mg)	From meal + cauliflower (No meat) (mg)
Vegetarian meal I	0.13	0.25 (meat)	0.32
Vegetarian meal II	0.13	0.44 (fish)	0.32
Vegetarian meal + iron	0.98	1.42 (meat)	—

The effect of fibre is important in nutritional terms because fibre intake is on the increase and indeed is actively encouraged by many nutritional and medical practitioners because of its alleged effect against constipation and its prophylaxis against some clinical conditions. If it does indeed have a deleterious effect on mineral absorption then in some cases, e.g. iron, calcium, and zinc, this action will exacerbate a situation that is already of concern to nutritionists and doctors. On the positive side, however, it must be remembered that high-fibre foods are usually exposed to the minimum of refining and processing and so retain most of their minerals, including iron. In addition, high-fibre supplements like bran are very rich in minerals.

Many studies on human beings involving dietary additions of wheat bran have failed to find a significant effect upon iron absorption at levels of bran up to 22g per day. Higher levels of wheat bran have yielded conflicting results. On one side Van Dokkum *et al.* reported in the *British Journal of Nutrition* in 1982 that 35g bran per day decreased iron absorption. Conversely E. Morris in 1983 in *Federation Proceedings* showed that more iron was assimilated when taken with 36g bran.

Studies on other high-fibre foods showed no effect. Soya bean seeds at intakes of 21g per day did not impair iron absorption in human volunteers (T. Schweizer *et al.*, *American Journal of Nutrition* [1983]). The uptake of iron was not affected by the ingestion of 24g fibre per day in human studies — in this case fruit and vegetables were the source of dietary fibre.

In animals, different varieties of fibre have been shown to have no effect upon iron absorption. At two levels of wheat bran representing 7 per cent and 20 per cent of the diet there was no inhibition of iron absorption in pigs and in rats. Fibre from a variety of sources including wheat bran, corn bran, soy bran, oat hulls, and cellulose (the fibre of fruit and vegetables) did not alter the absorption of iron, even when fed at the 6 per cent level of the diet to chickens and dogs. There was a small effect with rice bran.

The villain of dietary fibre appears to be phytic acid. This forms insoluble complexes with dietary iron and these complexes cannot be absorbed. According to Drs K. Kobza and V. Steenblock of the University of Basle, writing in the *British Medical Journal*, phytic acid is the reason that iron from wholemeal bread is not absorbed as well as that from white bread. Their results confirmed that wholemeal bread significantly inhibited the absorption of non-haem iron. At the same time they suggested that over-enthusiastic consumption of bran e.g. in breakfast cereals, may increase the long-term risk of iron deficiency by inducing a negative balance (i.e. iron absorption is less than iron losses).

Wholemeal flour contains more iron than unsupplemented white flour. This is why white flour is fortified with iron to bring it up to the level of 80 per cent extraction flour. Hence despite levels of 3.8 to 3.9mg iron per 100g wholemeal flour compared to 1.0mg per 100g in supplemented white flour, the absorption of iron from each type of flour when made into bread is similar (i.e. 0.11mg per 100g from wholemeal and 0.09mg per 100g from white). However, as mentioned previously, the type of iron added to supplement that in white flour is so poorly absorbed that the figure from fortified flour is similar to that from the unfortified variety.

—————Effect of beverages upon————— iron absorption

Three different reports from three different parts of the world have shown quite conclusively that tea has a potent inhibitory effect on the absorption of non-haem iron (the medical journals *Gut* [1975]; *South African Journal of Medical Science* [1975] and *New England Journal of Medicine* [1979]). In the *Gut* study, it was demonstrated that iron absorption from a meal could be reduced by as much as 87 per cent when tea was included. Now, further studies reported in the *American Journal of Clinical Nutrition* in 1983 implicate coffee as another beverage that can reduce absorption.

The results were as follows: when water was given with a hamburger meal, 3.71 per cent of the non-haem iron was absorbed. When tea replaced water, absorption of the mineral fell to 1.32 per cent, representing a highly significant 64 per cent inhibition. When infused coffee was the drink taken with the meal, only 2.25 per cent of the non-haem iron was absorbed, indicating a 39 per cent decrease when compared with water.

When a semi-purified meal was the source of food, coffee had an even greater inhibitory effect on iron absorption than with the hamburger meal. Absorption was only 1.64 per cent, compared to 72 per cent from the standard hamburger meal. Instant coffee was even more deleterious than the infused variety, reducing iron uptake from a massive 83 per cent. When instant coffee was prepared stronger, a further 45 per cent drop in iron absorption occurred.

These results confirmed earlier experiments by Dr M. Layrisse *et al.* reported in the *American Journal of Clinical Nutrition* (1976). They studied the availability of ferrous sulphate-fortified sugar added to several beverages. The reason behind such a study is that in South American countries, iron fortification is often carried out by adding iron salts to sugar. What emerged was that absorption from iron-fortified sugar was reduced by 44 per cent in a meal containing vegetables, meat, and coffee compared to the meal without coffee. Also coffee with milk was found to be twice as inhibitory as black coffee, suggesting that milk may also contribute to this deleterious effect.

Tea is thought to influence iron absorption because it contains tannic acid, which combines with non-haem iron to form insoluble iron tannates that cannot be assimilated by the body. Coffee is likely to inhibit iron absorption by a different mechanism, as indicated by other studies. This is because the reduction in absorption is most marked when the coffee is taken with the meal or one hour later. Even after this time, a significant fraction of the meal is still in the stomach. The practice of coffee after a meal should therefore appear to be undesirable when iron uptake is considered.

One important factor in determining why tea and coffee have this inhibitory effect is possibly the formation of ferric iron by both beverages. As we have seen, ferric iron has limited bioavailability for absorption in human beings.

The findings that tea and coffee have this adverse effect on iron availability have important implications for iron nutrition throughout the world. In the UK, Australia, New Zealand, and other tea-drinking countries, older people tend to have very high intakes of tea, and indeed in many cases the beverage is a part of the staple diet. When tea is taken in conjunction with meals that have a high non-haem iron content and low haem iron content it is easy to imagine iron absorption being adversely affected and the chances of deficiency increased.

Coffee, on the other hand, is commonly consumed in countries where iron-deficient anaemia is prevalent anyway, and so the beverage exacerbates the problem. In these countries, sugar is often the vehicle for supplying extra iron to the population, but as we have seen, using this sugar to sweeten coffee negates its usefulness to the person drinking it. Regrettably, no matter what type the supplement is, the iron in it is affected adversely by coffee and tea. These findings suggest therefore that when considering adding iron to the foods of unwitting populations, the authorities must consider very carefully the most effective way of doing this, taking into account the dietary habits of those populations.

How, then, can we overcome the inhibitory actions of phytic acid in cereals and tannic acid in tea and coffee on our iron absorption? The answer may have been given by Dr L. Hallberg and his team at University of Göteburg, Sweden. In 1986 they reported in *Human Nutrition: Applied Nutrition* that they had studied 299 people using radioactive labelled iron. They concluded that whilst ascorbic acid improved the absorption of non-haem iron in different types of meal when these were eaten without high fibre intakes and beverages, the same vitamin was able to overcome the inhibitory effects of these two factors. Both pure ascorbic acid and vitamin-rich foods neutralized these inhibitory effects. Dr Hallberg recommends that each main meal should contain about 50mg ascorbic acid to maintain this desirable function.

CHAPTER 4

Treating and Preventing Iron Deficiency

There are three fundamental questions relevant to the potential harmful effects of iron-deficiency anaemia. The first relates to the athlete, particularly the female, where maximal performance capacity may not be achieved. The second concerns the worker whose survival depends on his labour output and his daily work productivity, both factors crucial in retaining his job, particularly in developing countries. The third question is related to a person's general sense of well-being or vitality, and throughout the world a reduction in these represents the most common of manifestations of iron-deficiency anaemia regardless of social or economic standing. There are many studies indicating that there are economic advantages relating to increased work productivity after iron treatment, especially in developing countries. There is also ample evidence for the clinical impression that generally people with iron-deficiency anaemia suffer from those two common symptoms, tiredness and weakness.

In theory there are a number of intervention techniques that may be employed in preventing and treating iron-deficiency anaemia in populations. The magnitude of the problem is such that within the World Health Organization an International Nutritional Anaemia Consultative Group (INACG) has been formed to stimulate co-ordination and exchange of information between the various agencies engaged in reducing iron deficiency. Approaches to this end are:

(1) Reduction of iron requirements by adequate family planning programmes and hookworm eradication. Sadly in those parts of the world where hookworm infestation is a problem, long-term eradication is seldom achieved because of difficulties in preventing reinfestation.

(2) Alteration of dietary habits with increased intake of foods stimulating iron absorption or a reduced intake of foods inhibiting absorption of the mineral. More research, however, is needed on the effect of various dietary factors and of different techniques in preparing meals that may lead to effective and feasible ways of improving iron nutrition.

(3) Iron fortification of the diet. This is the method of choice when (a) large segments of the population are iron-deficient (b) suitable iron-carrying food vehicles are available that can reach a major part of the population (c) compatible iron fortification preparations are available. In industrialized countries fortification is necessary to replace iron that is not eaten in the diet because of lower food intake due mainly to reduced energy expenditure. In developing countries fortification is needed because the usual diet is insufficient in both energy and nutrients, including iron. In addition, these diets tend to be composed mainly of foods with low iron bioavailability.

(4) Therapeutic supplementation with iron tablets has to be used when there is a large deficit to be made up in a relatively short time. This is necessary in pregnant women and in those with severe anaemia.

Points 1, 2, and 3 have already been dealt with in previous chapters. Let us now look at supplementation with iron both in treating anaemia and in preventing the condition developing.

————————Treatment of iron deficiency————————

The response of iron deficiency anaemia to treatment by iron replenishment is influenced by several factors. These include the cause and severity of the iron deficient state, the presence of other complicating illnesses and the ability of the individual to tolerate and absorb medicinal iron. Effective therapy is followed by an increased rate of production of red blood cells, with the increase proportional to the severity of the anaemia and to the amount of iron made available to the bone marrow where production takes place. The bone marrow can only produce new red blood cells if it is given the tools, namely, iron.

This fact was illustrated by a study reported in 1969 by R. S. Hillman and P. A. Henderson (*Journal of Clinical Investigation*). When normal volunteers were deliberately bled, the rate of red blood cell production (called erythropoiesis) was reduced to less than one-third of the normal rate when the iron content of the blood plasma dropped below 70μg per 100ml. Once the plasma iron level increased to between 75 and 100μg per 100ml after iron therapy, red blood cell production increased to more than three times the normal rate. If the rate of destruction of red blood cells increases, serum iron levels also increase and production of new red cells is enhanced accordingly. This is the built-in safety measure that protects against worsening of the anaemia.

Another important factor in determining response to oral iron therapy is the ability of the individual to tolerate and absorb the mineral. There are clear limits to the tolerance of the gastro-intestinal tract to iron. The small intestine regulates absorption and prevents the entry of overwhelming amounts of iron into the bloodstream. Hence this places a ceiling on how much iron can be provided to the body by oral presentation. In the person with moderate anaemia, maximal doses of oral iron will supply from 40 to 60mg of the mineral to the bone marrow, and this is sufficient for production of new red blood cells at a rate two or three times the norm. As we shall see later, iron preparations do differ in their absorbability, and improved absorption can often mean less iron need be given orally.

Once a response to oral iron is demonstrated, therapy should be continued until the haemoglobin level returns to normal. It is then usual for treatment to be extended in order to replenish iron stores. This may take a considerable time since the rate of absorption of iron by the intestine will decrease markedly as iron stores are reconstituted.

The type of iron used most frequently in medicinal therapy of iron deficiency is ferrous sulphate, mainly because it is the least expensive of iron salts. The ferrous form is chosen because iron in the ferrous state is at least three times better absorbed than ferric iron, and at high dosage, the discrepancy is greater. The type of ferrous sulphate is the hydrated salt, and this provides about 20 per cent of its weight as iron. Other commonly used preparations are ferrous asparate (provides 14.2 per cent iron); ferrous carbonate saccharated (24 per cent iron); ferrous citrate (23.8 per cent iron); ferrous fumarate (31.3 per cent iron); ferrous gluconate (12.5 per cent iron); ferrous glycine sulphate (17.8 per cent iron); ferrous lactate (19.4 per cent iron); ferrous orotate (15.2 per cent iron); ferrous oxalate (31.1 per cent iron); ferrous succinate (32.6 per cent iron); and ferrous tartrate (22.5 per cent iron). Recently an amino-acid chelated form of iron has become available (e.g. Aminochel iron), which provides 10 per cent of its weight as iron.

The usual therapeutic dose of iron is about 200mg per day (i.e. 2 to 3mg per kg body weight), so the actual amount of the iron preparation needed depends upon its percentage of iron. Hence a dose is usually given as 60mg iron three times daily. Children weighing 15 to 30kg can take half the adult dose. Smaller children and infants are able to tolerate larger doses of iron than adults, so their usual dosage is 5mg per kg body weight. It must be stressed that these dosages are for the treatment of iron-deficiency anaemia and should not be regarded as prophylactic or supplementary doses to prevent anaemia. When the object is the prevention of iron deficiency, e.g. in pregnant women, doses of 15 to 30mg per day are adequate to meet the 3 to 6mg daily requirements of the last six months of pregnancy.

Absorption of iron is optimal when the ferrous salts are taken on an empty stomach. This is because there are factors in food which may reduce the availability of an iron salt. It has been shown that the bioavailability of iron salts ingested with food is probably only one-half to one-third that seen in the fasted subject. Even though taking ferrous salts on an empty stomach may increase the chances of gastro-intestinal distress, it is claimed by some that it is preferable to reduce the dose in these circumstances than to take the iron with food. These considerations apply to ferrous salts. There is now increasing evidence that iron taken in the form of amino-acid chelates or other chelates (i.e. gluconates) are better absorbed than iron salts with or without food.

Small doses of iron taken a number of times daily are preferred to single, high-potency doses even if they are of the so-called timed or sustained release types. This is because low doses are absorbed better, and taken frequently will maintain high blood plasma concentrations of iron. This is illustrated in Table 18.

Such figures are average and may be modified by the severity of the iron-deficiency anaemia and by the presence or absence of food, but they do indicate that to triple the amount of iron

Table 18 Absorption and response to oral iron

Total dose mg/day	Estimated absorption %	mg	Haemoglobin increase g/100ml blood
35	40	14	0.07
105	24	25	0.14
195	18	35	0.19
390	12	45	0.22

actually absorbed, the total intake must increase eleven-fold. This high intake must enhance the chances of side-effects, and regular and frequent low-dose ingestion is usually preferred.

Supplementation with iron

We have seen that in foods, haem iron is absorbed far more efficiently than non-haem iron even when the latter is assisted by vitamin C. The absorption of iron from iron salts is comparable to that of non-haem iron and vitamin C can help here also. The difference between the positive effect of the vitamin on food, non-haem iron, and iron salts is in the amount of vitamin C needed to effect better absorption. In a meal, this can be as little as 50mg (see above), but when taken with iron salts, more of the vitamin is needed.

Professor L. Hallberg and his colleagues (e.g. H. Brize and L. Hallberg, *Acta. Med. Scand.* [1962]) have shown in a number of published studies that at least 200mg ascorbic acid is needed to increase the absorption of iron from iron salts by 30 per cent. It is essential that both vitamins and minerals are taken together. The same studies indicated that in some people, this enhanced absorption is sufficient to increase the chances and incidence of side-effects due to excess iron. Hence the sensible approach if you wish to ensure good absorption of iron from iron salts by taking extra vitamin C is to keep the potency of the iron down to reasonable quantities, i.e. not more than 24mg of the mineral at any one time. This amount is the maximum iron per unit dose allowed by the DHSS in licensed products containing iron for general sale to the public (the medicines, general sale list order 1984, SI No. 769).

The ideal supplement is one that is identical to or related closely to haem iron since this is the best-absorbed type of iron regardless of vitamin C. Whilst no one has produced a haem iron supplement (except for dried blood or haemoglobin, which vegetarians and vegans will not accept), the nearest approach to it is the amino-acid chelated mineral. What, then do 'chelation' and 'mineral chelates' mean?

————Chelated iron and other minerals————

The term 'chelation' covers a number of processes, and we have to distinguish between chelation in the chemical and in the biological sense. If a person is poisoned with heavy metals such as lead or mercury, a compound such as ethylenediaminetetracetic acid (EDTA)—or, in case of copper poisoning, d-penicillamine— is often injected into the individual, the reason being that these compounds chelate the minerals, producing a very stable compound that is easily excreted and is non-toxic. At the other end of the scale there are so-called weak chelates such as ascorbates, lactates, and citrates, where the metal is bound to a residue which, although chemically speaking is a chelate, is no more stable than inorganic salts—in fact as food supplements these chelates are just as inefficient. Gluconates are chelates where the mineral is bound up with the natural sugar residue gluconic acid, and these look from recent studies to be better absorbed than mineral (including iron) salts. The true biological chelate consists of a mineral surrounded by amino-acids. Amino-acids are the units that go to make up the proteins, and in the body every mineral, apart from the skeletal minerals calcium and phosphorus, is present as an amino-acid or a protein chelate. If this were not so, life would be impossible because the injection of inorganic metal salts directly into the blood system produces gross toxic effects and eventually death.

A chelated mineral may be regarded as essentially a mineral completely surrounded by amino-acids. It can be imagined as a ball-bearing, which represents the mineral or metal, surrounded by a ball of clay, representing the amino-acids. If you can picture this, you can see how well the ball-bearing would be protected if it were thrown, if it were passed through something, even if it were mixed with some sort of food; you can imagine how the ball of clay would stay intact, all the time protecting the essential ball-bearing in the centre of it. Another important point is that the ball of clay is composed of amino-acids, which means that the digestive processes of the body are not going to attack it in any way, because their ultimate function, of course, is to produce amino-acids, and here we have them already. Typical examples of natural chelates are iron in haemoglobin, magnesium in chlorophyll, zinc in insulin, calcium in milk, chromium and selenium in yeast, and cobalt in vitamin B12.

The idea of producing iron chelated with amino-acids to mimic haem iron as far as possible has been around for many years and much research has gone into ways and means of making such chelates in the laboratory. Before the advent of amino-acid chelated minerals (including iron) the combination of the minerals with intact protein was tried and the resulting complex showed promise in better absorption of the mineral compared to that of mineral salts when incorporated into farm animal feeds. All sorts of protein were tried but for commercial reasons fish was usually the source. Of course, as we have seen, even the presence of fish, meat, and poultry in a meal can enhance non-haem iron absorption, but the extra iron absorbed from proteinates and even more so from amino-acid chelates appears to outweigh this in experiments conducted so far.

Much of the research into how minerals are absorbed has been carried out by Albion Laboratories of Utah, USA over the last thirty years. What they have done is to take the minerals and chelate them with amino-acids, themselves produced from soya protein, reproducing in the laboratory as close as is possible what nature has done in foods. It is particularly significant that their research has shown that the chelates produced using their potential processes are absorbed into the intestinal cells intact. You may recall that it is at this stage that there is the essential difference between haem iron and non-haem iron. Haem iron (and amino acid chelated iron) does not have to have the complexing ligand removed before absorption, but non-haem and iron salts do. Once inside the intestinal cell, both types of iron end up complexed to protein and amino acids within that cell and are then transferred to the bloodstream in a similar way. The amino acid chelated minerals produced by Albion Laboratories are available throughout the UK and other countries under the trade name *Aminochels*.

Having established that it is possible to create an animo acid chelate of a mineral in a similar fashion to that of Nature, how do we know that these particular minerals are better absorbed? The techniques used involve radioactive tracer minerals — minerals with a radioactive charge on them incorporated into an amino acid chelate that can be traced inside an animal or, in some cases, man, proving conclusively that this particular mineral has been absorbed. Using such techniques, absorption of minerals presented in different forms can be studied both in isolated jejunum (the part of the small intestine where minerals are mainly absorbed) and in intact animals.

Typical results from such experiments are as follows; in each case the ratio of iron absorbed from iron amino acid chelate to that from conventional iron supplements is quoted:

Iron amino acid chelate/ferrous carbonate 3.6:1
Iron amino acid chelate/ferrous sulphate 3.8:1
Iron amino acid chelate/ferrous oxide 4.9:1

In every case, absorption of iron from the amino acid chelate is superior to that from other forms of the mineral.

Similar experiments in pigs, cows and poultry carried out at Albion Laboratories and fully reported in the literature indicate the superiority of the absorption of iron from the amino-acid chelate. Pigs are of particular importance because a serious problem in new-born piglets is lack of iron, causing life-threatening anaemia. One reason for this is the poor transference of iron across the placenta from sow to piglets whilst they are developing. The standard treatment for the problem is an injection of iron into each piglet when born in an attempt to overcome the iron deficiency before this becomes fatal. It has been shown that feeding the sow amino-acid chelated iron before farrowing enables her iron levels to build up to such an extent that sufficient mineral can cross the placenta and be deposited in the piglets. At present, most of the iron amino-acid chelates produced by Albion find their way into animal feeds, but more recent research has indicated that human beings too can benefit from increased iron absorption from these supplements.

Amino-acid chelated iron in human anaemia

One clinical trial was carried out by Dr H. Schruffers of the University of Augsburg, Bavaria. Sixteen anaemic patients were treated with iron in the amino-acid chelated form (Aminochel brand) for a period of three weeks. Patients numbered from 1 to 6 received 48mg iron daily (i.e. six Aminochel tablets). Those numbered from 7 to 16 received 64mg iron daily (i.e. eight Aminochel tablets). In all cases, the levels of haemoglobin, red blood cells, and serum iron were measured in each patient before treatment started and after it had finished. The results were as follows:

HAEMOGLOBIN LEVEL	Cases 1 to 6	10% increase
	Cases 7 to 16	18.9% increase
	Average	14.4% increase
RED BLOOD CELL COUNT	Cases 1 to 6	19% increase
	Cases 7 to 16	15.2% increase
	Average	12.1% increase
SERUM IRON VALUE	Cases 1 to 6	49% increase
	Cases 7 to 16	80% increase
	Average	64.5% increase

Dr Schruffers reported that the compatibility and acceptability of the tablets were very good. The only side-effects noted were two cases of mild diarrhoea which in his opinion were due to nutritional factors not associated with the iron supplement.

A more comprehensive clinical trial on similar tablets was carried out by Professor H. W. Kirchhoff, Medical Director of the Sanatorium Nordrach, Augsburg, Bavaria. The subjects were 30 patients (19 male, 11 female) with a mean age of 46 years (range 35 to 68 years). All suffered from iron-deficiency anaemia induced by other conditions, e.g. haemorrhage from peptic ulcer, prostatic cancer operation, and ulcerative colitis in the males. In the females the anaemia was a result of hysterectomy with severe subsequent haemorrhage, Crohn's disease, and Hodgkin's disease. Crohn's disease is of interest since a feature is often decreased absorption of nutrients. In addition, the following risk-factors were present in some of the patients: diabetes mellitus, hyperlipidaemia, obesity, and heavy smoking.

The therapeutic phase lasted for 28 days. Daily throughout the four weeks of therapy one Aminochel iron tablet (containing 8mg iron) was ingested each morning, midday, and evening to provide a total supplementary intake of 24mg iron. Care was taken to ensure that the tablets were always taken before meals at the same hour of the day. Blood samples were taken before the trial started and at the end of each week of therapy. Many tests were carried out, but those that concern us are the haemoglobin, red blood cell count, serum iron, and haematocrit tests.

Symptoms of side-effects

A daily record was compiled of the following clinical symptoms — lassitude, fatigue, lower chest pressure, gastric pain (cutting, burning, and cramp-like), sense of fullness, belching, nausea, vomiting, and any other symptoms. The scale used was intense, present, or absent.

Evaluation

Minimum value, maximum value, arithmetic mean value, and standard deviation were all calculated for the four parameters serum iron, red cell count, haemoglobin, and haematocrit.

Results

All these parameters increased significantly during the period of therapy. Even after one week a slight but significant therapeutic effect was noted. The response of the various patients was not uniform, but this is to be expected. In terms of absolute increases, these were as follows:

Serum iron increased from   41.2 to 65.3 $\mu g/100ml$
Red cell count increased from   3.55 to   4.17 $\times 10^6/cmm$
Haemoglobin increased from   10.88 to 12.49 $g/100ml$
Haematocrit increased from   32.11 to 37.32%

Side-effects

All patients tolerated the tablets well, and there were no gastro-intestinal symptoms reported. In none of the side-effects was the level 'strongly present' reported. Gastric pain (45 occasions), sense of fullness (16 occasions), and constipation (8 occasions) were reported, but only at the 'present' level. All three side-effects occurred most frequently at the start of medication. As the four parameters increased, so did the incidence of side-effects decrease. None of the other parameters measured changed during the trial, indicating that tolerance to the treatment was high with no biochemical side-effects.

————Conclusion by Professor Kirchhoff————

Amino-acid chelated iron effectively increases haematopoiesis (i.e. blood formation) but with very few side-effects. During the relatively short trial of four weeks, all the patients' parameters returned to their normal range. Particularly noteworthy are the following findings:

> Therapeutic response occurs in only a few days; there is a marked effect upon the patients' general condition and liveliness; side-effects are few; the product is of practical application . . . There is obviously a high rate of absorption. No serious side-effects were encountered. No other parameters were changed, indicating lack of biochemical side-effects.

Further studies using radioactive iron to determine absorption and bioavailability and to measure serum ferritin levels were suggested, and these are at present awaiting official approval.

In neither trial was it possible to compare in the same patient response to amino-acid chelate with that of conventional iron therapy, which of course is well established. However, the following table provides a comparison of iron (as chelate) in the trial with iron (as various other preparations) used in conventional treatment.

Form of iron	Iron per day
Ferrous sulphate	120–80mg
Ferrous aspatate	142–213mg
Ferrous fumarate	130–95mg
Ferrous gluconate	144–92mg
Iron amino-acid chelate	24mg

With the other iron preparations haemoglobin may take up to 10 weeks to reach normal values. The increase starts at the end of 2 weeks, but thereafter the haemoglobin should rise by 0.7–1g/100ml weekly.

In the case of iron amino-acid chelate a response was noted after one week and normal levels were reached after four weeks.

A third clinical trial in which the absorption of iron from iron amino-acid chelate was compared with that from ferrous sulphate in 12 individual patients was carried out at the Mount Sinai School of Medicine, Mount Sinai Medical Center, New York, USA. In addition, however, the effect of 250mg of vitamin C on the absorption of iron from the chelate was also researched. The results are shown in Table 19.

Table 19 Iron absorption study (all subjects received 18mg elemental iron)

Patient		Iron % absorbed		
Age	Sex	Ferrous sulphate	Aminochel iron	Chelate plus vitamin C
45	M	5.0	11.1	16.2
33	F	8.2	14.0	18.0
27	F	18.1	21.0	28.9
24	M	9.0	12.2	13.9
53	F	11.1	16.1	19.0
60	M	8.4	13.0	20.9
53	M	11.0	16.0	24.0
49	M	6.1	14.2	30.8
36	F	14.3	19.0	28.0
53	M	7.3	13.1	19.2
58	M	5.2	12.0	23.0
61	F	12.1	18.0	26.0

The average absorption of iron from ferrous sulphate was 9.5 per cent; that from iron amino-acid chelate 15.1 per cent (i.e. 59 per cent better than from ferrous sulphate), and that from iron amino-acid chelate plus vitamin C 22.3 per cent (i.e. 125 per cent better than from ferrous sulphate).

It has been established that vitamin C does not enhance the absorption of haem iron, so the fact that the vitamin increases the absorption of iron from Aminochel iron would suggest that the form of the mineral in this preparation is not identical with that in haem. Nevertheless, the significant improvement in the absorption of the mineral from the chelate compared to that from ferrous sulphate proves that the iron is inferior to the mineral in the sulphate as far as absorption is concerned. Perhaps it is somewhere in structure between ferrous salts and iron in haem when present in the chelate.

Studies are at present under way to produce an iron chelate that is nearer to haem iron in structure so as to increase the extent of absorption even further. Until then, however, iron amino-acid chelate remains the best form of absorbed iron that is available at present.

────Clinical trials with ferrous gluconate────

Ferrous gluconate has been used as a source of iron for therapeutic as well as prophylactic purposes for at least 50 years. In 1937, Drs O. Peznikoff and W. F. Goebel reported in the *Journal of Clinical Investigation* that daily intakes of 108 to 216mg iron as the gluconate cured iron-deficiency anaemia in thirteen female parties ranging in age from 24 to 49 years. They noted that the response to oral ferrous gluconate was so good that there was no real advantage in giving the supplement in injectable form. They were pleased to note that those patients who had experienced side-effects with other iron preparations were able to take ferrous gluconate without any undue distress.

In another trial carried out by Dr D. Haler in 1952 and reported in the *British Medical Journal* of that year, ferrous gluconate, providing 105mg iron daily, along with vitamins including vitamin C was given to a group of anaemic patients. The period of treatment required to raise the haemoglobin value to normal was only 17.8 days on average in these patients. 'The liquid ferrous gluconate preparation was far and away the most popular with patients and produced a therapeutic response out of all expectations', reported Dr Haler.

In another trial reported in the *Journal of Laboratory and Clinical Medicine* in 1952 (M. R. Gram and R. M. Leverton) the absorption of iron from ferrous gluconate was compared to that from ferrous lactate and ferrous sulphate in daily intakes of 100mg of the mineral on the basis of haematological response. There was no significant difference in the amount of iron absorbed from all three preparations, but the incidence of side-effects was lowest in those receiving ferrous gluconate.

We can conclude therefore that in human studies ferrous gluconate proved to be a very effective presentation of iron in the therapy of iron-deficiency anaemia with the distinct advantage of causing less distress in the individual than iron salts.

Side-effects of iron therapy

Intolerance to oral preparations of iron is primarily a function of the amount of soluble iron in the upper part of the gastro-intestinal tract and of psychological factors. The latter often weigh more heavily than many people imagine. Common side-effects include heartburn, nausea, upper gastric discomfort, constipation, and diarrhoea. If there has been a previous intolerance to iron, it is sound policy to start therapy at a small dosage that does not give rise to symptoms and gradually increase the intake to that desired.

The usual therapeutic dose is 200mg iron per day in three divided doses, and at this level approximately 25 per cent of individuals suffer some side-effects, compared with 13 per cent amongst those receiving a placebo. At high dosage the usual complaints are nausea and abdominal pain. On the other hand constipation and diarrhoea, possibly related to the effect of iron on the bacteria that inhabit the lower gut, are no more prevalent at high dosage than at lower intakes. Heartburn is no worse either.

Chronic iron overload

Toxic effects due to long-term administration of iron can occur and give rise to the condition of haemochromatosis according to case-studies reported by Dr T. H. Bothwell *et al., Iron Metabolism in Man* (Blackwell, 1979). In this condition, massive amounts of iron in the storage forms ferritin and haemosiderin are laid down in body tissues. Available evidence suggests that the normal person is able to control absorption of iron, but this control appears to be missing in those who are prone to haemochromatosis. In other words haemochromatosis is usually the result of some genetic failure.

Iron thus gradually builds up in the body, so it is usually middle age before symptoms of genetically induced haemochromatosis appear. Large amounts of fibrous tissue form in many organs, leading to enlarged liver with cirrhosis, pancreatic diabetes, and a slate-grey discoloration of the skin. Iron is deposited in the pituitary gland and this in time affects the sexual glands, causing a reduction in secretion and size. Haemochromatosis can eventually be fatal if steps are not taken to remove the excess iron from the body.

Other reasons for iron overload, but much rarer, include haemolytic anaemia, where there is excessive destruction of red blood cells. The iron released is then deposited outside the usual storage depots because they become saturated with the mineral. Repeated blood transfusions can also lead to iron overload when the iron excretion mechanisms break down. There is at least one case on record of a man whose content of iron was so high due to long-term therapy and blood transfusions that he was able to trigger off the security metal detectors at an airport!

Excessive nutritional intakes

Overload due to eating too much iron from the food or from supplements is more common and is known as siderosis. It can happen with prolonged intakes of over 40mg iron daily. The commonest cause is iron contamination from vessels used in cooking and in producing alcoholic beverages. The classic case is that of the Bantu population of Johannesburg, South Africa, who drink beer brewed from maize or sorghum in iron vessels. Most of our knowledge of iron overload comes from studying these people (e.g. D. P. Derman et al., British Journal of Nutrition [1980]).

Other reports have come from Boston, USA (R. A. McDonald 1964) of siderosis amongst the poor wine-drinking population of that city. Cheap wines can contain up to 40mg iron per litre compared to the more usual 10mg per litre in the better varieties. Rough and home-produced cider produced in iron vessels can also provide as much as 16mg iron per litre, so the intake of large volumes of the beverage can lead to nutritional iron overload. These high intakes are common in the diet of such people, but anyone who takes daily supplements of iron above 40mg for prolonged periods may also be prone to overload, although manifestations may not appear for many years.

Assessment of iron overload in a population is usually made by measurements of iron storage in the livers at post-mortem. By this means it has become apparent that the problem is decreasing in the Johannesburg population where it was prevalent. One reason is the switch from home-brewed beer to the commercial variety. However, in other communities in Africa the problem is still present because iron cooking pots are very much in use. Whilst a mild degree of overload is probably harmless, there is some evidence that it can be a contributory factor in the development of liver cirrhosis.

Iron poisoning

Large amounts of ferrous salts, particularly ferrous sulphate, are toxic, but in adults fatalities are rare and almost always suicidal. Children, however, can easily be poisoned with iron salts, and as little as 3 grams of ferrous sulphate can cause death in a small child. In most fatal cases, though, the amount ingested is nearer 10 grams. The high frequency of iron poisoning relates to its availability in the average household and tends to occur in those where there is or has been a pregnancy since it is then that ferrous salts tend to be present in the house. The moral is obvious — all iron preparations must be kept out of the reach of children, particularly as the tablets are often sugar-coated and in attractive colours.

Signs and symptoms of acute iron poisoning may occur within 30 minutes or be delayed for several hours depending upon stomach contents. There is usually severe abdominal pain and diarrhoea and/or vomiting of brown or bloody stomach contents. Of particular concern are pallor or bluish colouration of the skin, lassitude, and drowsiness, since these symptoms are usually the forerunners of cardio-vascular collapse.

If death does not occur within 6 hours there may be a transient period of apparent recovery, but death can still happen in 12 to 24 hours. Hence in any case of suspected acute iron salt poisoning, professional help should be sought as soon as possible. The value of this is reflected in the mortality rate of iron poisoning in children, which has been reduced from 45 per cent in the past to about 1 per cent at the present time.

Index